UNDER THE BUCKEYE TREE

The gifts, frustrations and
challenges of Multiple Sclerosis

Keith & Dare Ford

Mountain Page Press
HENDERSONVILLE, NC

Editor: Brenda Dammann
Cover design: Daniel Ojedokun

DEDICATION

This book is dedicated to the many individuals diagnosed with an illness that has changed the direction of their lives, dreams, and goals. And to the caregivers who are faithfully devoted to their care with love and support.

Life can bring many changes and challenges in a moment. It takes faith and courage to discover the inner strength to cope.

May those who find themselves in this situation be blessed with encouragement and peace in their lives.

ACKNOWLEDGEMENTS

Thank you to Mr. Gene Weller, the artist who kindly drew the image of the buckeye tree for the title of this book. We met Gene 40-some years ago in Asheville, North Carolina. He, along with his wife, Mary, and daughter, attended the same church. Mary started the daycare center at church that our daughter, Elizabeth, and son, Andrew, attended. After Gene and Mary moved, we lost communication for several years. However, we later reconnected, and during a visit talked with Gene about our desire to write this book. Through our conversations, Gene agreed to draw the cover. We appreciate his undertaking and the art.

Recognition goes to Chandler Ragsdale, who supported and encouraged the original organization of this manuscript. We first met when Chandler was attending Southern Wesleyan University and working as youth minister at our church. We met frequently over the months to discuss ideas and recommendations regarding this story.

Thank you to Marian Godwin, Doris Johnson, and Ann Cason for their continued support, encouragement, and friendship. All three have assisted us in the completion of this project.

Special love to our children Elizabeth and Andrew who have both been by my side in this journey.

Particular acknowledgement goes to those individuals who suffer from an illness or condition requiring strength and courage to battle each day. Their struggles highlight the need for further medical research and interventions that can prevent, help, or cure disease.

And lastly, a we s... those caregivers who give of themselves to assist and address the needs of loved ones. Through their care, dedication, and compassion they provide faith, hope, and encouragement.

TABLE OF CONTENTS

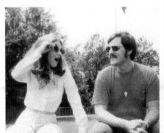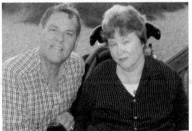

CHALLENGES

This is a journey that extends over a period of 45 years. It covers the time from our first meeting in 1975 to the present day and tells a story of our love, dedication, and devotion through sickness and health. It has been 25 years since Dare's 1995 medical diagnosis. As her health has declined, her needs for care have increased, and my role as husband has changed to include that of caretaker.

It's been challenging to balance the two.

Our goal is to share our connection, discuss the challenges and frustrations faced, and reveal the gifts encountered along the way.

LESSON LEARNED

Dare:

As a person with a progressive and chronic illness, I've received many blessings and positive gifts. I've been touched by strangers who helped me and those who prayed for me. My biggest gift, however, comes from a husband who stays with me when he could easily give up. My faith and family continue to sustain me. I don't worry about the future because I've received the gift of learning to live in the present moment. I appreciate the things given me every day.

Keith:

As a primary caregiver, I'm learning to meet the challenges of this role. Caregiving is demanding. There are moments of isolation, frustration, and anger. I have learned that this emotional roller coaster is normal. Although I've struggled at times with the challenges,

I've also been successful recognizing the strengths and positive qualities within me that enable me to continue providing care: maintaining her safety, meeting her medical needs, providing her nutritional care, and addressing her daily activities of living. Above it all, my love for her remains my primary focus.

MULTIPLE SCLEROSIS

Multiple Sclerosis is a disabling disease of the brain and central nervous system where the immune system attacks the myelin (the protective sheath covering the nerve fibers), creating communication problems between the brain and other areas of the body. It's an autoimmune disease, meaning the immune system mistakenly attacks various tissues or organs of the body. There is no known cause of MS, and while research suggests genetic factors may increase risk, there is no direct evidence that MS is inherited.

Diagnosis is often hard to confirm, and symptoms of the disorder can vary from individual to individual. Magnetic resonance imaging (MRI) is often utilized to search for evidence of lesions in the brain and spinal cord, which helps to make the diagnosis.

There are different categories of MS. Some patients experience relapsing-remitting MS, where the disease causes a temporary increase in symptoms by attacking the body's immune system before retreating again. The patient can often return to normal, or near-normal, physical activities between attacks.

Other patients experience chronic and secondary progressive MS, which causes devastating and lasting impairment over time. This type of MS creates a permanent deterioration of function that does not return. Symptoms can result in a loss of mental function in addition to physical impairment.

There are several medications which can slow the progression and symptoms of MS, but no one medication has successfully reversed or stopped the disease.

UNDER THE BUCKEYE TREE

Each of us has a story to tell, a journey of experiences.

Our story is no different.

In our relationship, we've dealt with the death of a daughter and concerns for our surviving children. We have experienced moments of loss, love, and acceptance. This story shares our journey, experiences, and hopes while also providing encouragement to those who face challenges in life.

The book title, *Under the Buckeye Tree*, has special meaning for us. As we strolled the sidewalks toward our town, we would pass a local high school in the center and stop to rest under the shade of a large buckeye tree with limbs that stretched across a portion of the campus. There was a wooden bench directly under her base. I would push Dare's wheelchair under the tree, close to this bench, and we would have private talks.

Sometimes the focus would be on our children, their activities, and their schoolwork. Other times the subject would be our careers, relationship, or her medical concerns and needs. Whatever the topic, the tree offered us a safe place to share intimate moments. I would often lie down and look up between the leaves and limbs to view the clouds floating against a brilliant blue sky. We cherished this time, sitting quietly in the stillness offered by the tree, before continuing our walk toward town and back home.

Sometimes one might find me walking alone to the buckeye tree just to think, write, or sit in quietness, organizing my thoughts and prayers for strength and faith. Under her shade I received moments of peace and solitude, slowing the questions of the mind.

Since the formulation of this book, the buckeye tree has been removed to make room for a new renovation to the high school. However, we will always treasure the gifts *under the buckeye tree* for giving us an intimate place to share thoughts and search for answers, truth, and understanding.

CHAPTER 1

OUR INITIAL MEETING

Keith:

It was a brisk fall afternoon as I stood on the porch of my mom and dad's home. Looking out toward the mountain tops, I saw the apple orchard that surrounded their property. The trees were laden with ripe apples drooping heavily toward the ground. Soon trucks would arrive to haul the produce to the juice factory.

The half mile driveway wound through the orchard to their house on the hill. On a dry day, dust would fly up over the treetops as vehicles approached. I recognized a car rounding the final curve before parking at the front steps. It was my sister, Kathy, and her boyfriend, Charlie.

Dare:

As Charlie turned the curve leading to Kathy's parents' home, I saw a young man standing on the front porch. I asked, "Who is that?" Charlie, answered, "Oh, that's Kathy's brother, 'Keithie-bug.'"

I was quite surprised; I knew her brother had his own apartment and didn't live with his parents. It never crossed my mind that I might end up meeting him unexpectedly that weekend. I had forgotten that she wanted me to meet him.

When I first saw him, I realized he wasn't bad looking. He was a handsome, tall, dark-haired young man. He was dressed in a pinstripe shirt with colors of red, blue, yellow, and white, and wearing stylish blue jeans with white tennis shoes.

Keith:

Kathy and her boyfriend had come from Western Carolina University for a long weekend visit. I forgot that Kathy was supposed to participate in the Apple Festival parade, part of the annual celebration honoring the county's apple business. Hendersonville's Main Street comes alive with crafts, art, and food vendors. In the evenings children and adults spontaneously dance to the music played in front of the old county courthouse. On Monday, the parade proceeds down Main Street with decorated floats, bands, and antique cars. There were beauty queens, politicians, and local law enforcement vehicles. My sister was to ride a float of a relative's furniture company.

The car door opened and Kathy jumped out with a big smile. After speaking to both her and Charlie, I realized there was a third individual in the back seat of the car. As she stepped out, the afternoon sunshine highlighted her vibrant red hair and a face glowing with a warm smile. Kathy introduced her as a college friend she had invited to watch her ride in the parade. Dare said, "I've heard a lot about you," and I responded, "I hope it was all good!" She assured me it was.

I learned later that Kathy had invited Dare home several times. She wanted her to meet me, but Dare was reluctant, fearing that if a blind date didn't work it would disrupt her relationship with Kathy. We always told Dare that the weekend was a setup, and that I had intentionally been waiting to meet her. She has never learned the truth to this story, and neither Kathy nor I have ever told her!

As the afternoon continued, the two of us engaged in long discussion, sharing and learning more about each other. Dare relayed that she had taken a year-long internship teaching seventh graders at Waynesville Junior High School, choosing this position over student teaching. She would start the next week and be given a year's teaching credit along with half of a salary. She had rented an apartment at Lake Junaluska Methodist Convention Center, which included a large lake surrounded by scenic mountain ranges in Waynesville, North Carolina.

I shared that I had graduated from Western Carolina University with a bachelor's degree in psychology. I was presently employed with Hendersonville's city school system as a counselor working with all levels of students K-12. Our love of children in a school setting was a common bond.

As we spent time together I was struck by this attractive, smart, goal-driven, energetic woman. She appeared to know who she was and where she was headed. I was taken by her smile, warm personality, and confidence.

Dare:

I was reared on a chicken farm in the North Carolina Piedmont. This was a small community town of Lilesville, near Wadesboro, where my father sold chickens and eggs to the community. I was the third of five children, with two older brothers and one three years younger. I was the only girl until my sister was born when I was ten years old. I was in fifth grade at that time and grew up with brothers who were extremely competitive. Not wanting to be called a "sissy" by my brothers because I was a "girl," I often participated in challenges that proved I was as capable.

For example, while in high school, I applied to drive a school bus, a rare activity for a girl. I knew I could do a "man's" job. The school personnel gave me this job not realizing that "Dare" was a girl's name, not a boy's name! I drove the bus for two years just to show my brothers I was as good as they.

When 16 years old, I was selected to attend a summer enrichment program for gifted students at Western Carolina University. While at Western, I fell in love with the mountains and decided it was where I wanted to complete my undergraduate studies.

During my college years, I had an opportunity to study in London, England for a semester and toured several of the European countries by myself. My parents were always supportive of my determination to accomplish my goals.

Keith:

I shared that I was the third child born in Hendersonville, NC. I had two brothers who were five years and three years older. When I turned 3½, a sister came into our lives. We grew up in the Catholic faith and attended the local Catholic school until seventh grade. Faith and service were most important.

Dare:

That night, we sat with his parents at the family dining table for an evening meal. Keith said he was on a diet and trying to quit smoking. He only ate grapes while the rest of us had a regular meal.

His mom said, "I'm looking for someone to take him off our hands. They need to be Irish, Catholic, and a Democrat!" I said, "Well, I'm two out of the three!"

Laughingly, she said, "Well that's good enough. Let me get his laundry ready for you." I thought that was funny because I knew he didn't even live there.

After the meal, I really enjoyed sitting in the living room with Keith, sharing a conversation. At one point he said, "Will you please excuse me? I need to make a quick phone call." He left and returned saying, "I was supposed to meet some family friends for the parade on Monday, but thought I would rather go with you, Charlie, and Kathy."

Keith:

We spent the entire evening in my parents living room talking and sharing our goals and aspirations. It was an extremely enjoyable time, and her company was comfortable. The next few days were spent attending the events of the holiday and watching the parade on Labor Day before she returned to her apartment. Whether it was the timing, circumstances, or stars in the sky…it was an amazing and magical weekend.

Dare:

Monday morning, Kathy braided my hair in pigtails. She and I acted silly, laughing and singing a kids song called "Little Rabbit Foo Foo" before going to the parade. It was an enjoyable afternoon, and soon it was time for us to return to Waynesville for school the next day.

I left the weekend with no expectations of seeing him again. On Tuesday afternoon, we stopped by the post office to check our mail. I was so surprised to receive a letter from Keith, telling me he enjoyed the weekend and wanted to come over for a ballgame between our two schools. I thought he was a nice guy, but never expected a letter so soon. I was surprised that he took the time to write that quickly.

He came, as promised, for a double date with Kathy and Charlie for the ballgame. We had such a good time and began seeing each other on weekends.

I was enthralled with him. He was a perfect gentleman and more mature than most guys I had dated in college. He impressed me with his kindness, respect, and manners. I appreciated the fact that he wasn't too forward and respected my moral values of no premarital sex. I knew he was attracted to my heart and personality, not just looks.

I will never forget our first kiss. We were sitting on a stone wall one night near my apartment. I had a fireball candy in my mouth when he asked for a kiss. I said, "Yes." I was so excited.

We spent the next eight months dating and enjoying each other. Keith was always romantic and would pick flowers for me during our walks. On the weekends, when I went to Hendersonville, Keith would never let me leave for home unless he gave me money for gas or in the event of car trouble. He was so concerned for my safety.

Once, when we shared childhood memories, Keith told a story of having a pack of gum and chewing the entire pack. I said, "When my mom gave me gum, it was half a stick for each kid." Keith said, "You poor little thing." I spoke up and said, "I was a rich little poor girl." I was happy with half a stick and Keith was a poor little rich boy who had a whole pack of gum for himself and was still not happy. We would tease each other as we recognized these differences in our childhood.

Keith was privileged to grow up with more material things than I. My dad would always say, "You need to know the difference between a want and a need." We always had plenty of food and comfort in our home, but never much extra. Keith had several school outfits from the Belk department store. My mother made most of my school clothes or I received hand-me-downs from an older cousin. Occasionally, Mom would buy me a new dress for Easter or when starting the school year.

Keith:

Fall was a beautiful time to date around Lake Junaluska, where she lived. This was an intimate location, where we spent time building a relationship and sharing our dreams. We would spend weekend afternoons walking around the lake, feeding the ducks, and talking of our goals and love of each other's company. One special afternoon, I suggested that we have a picnic. I arranged her dining room table on her driveway, and we enjoyed an evening in the fall air.

On another occasion, Dare and I went to a football game at my school. She had just had her hair cut and wore a sexy red dress with a stylish black coat. As we entered the stadium, several of my school students yelled out,

"Mr. Ford, you've got a beautiful woman! She must be your girlfriend!" I felt so proud, not only being with a beautiful woman, but one who shared many of the qualities I was searching for. The night was special, she looked wonderful, and we won the ballgame! What an exceptional time!

Dare and I loved music, especially the songs of John Denver. One day we took a drive to the mountaintop known as "Jump Off Rock." It was a cool fall afternoon, and the view of the mountains was fabulous. I took my guitar along and tried to play a song by John Denver. Dare listened as I sang "Sunshine On My Shoulders." Later, Dare surprised me with a shirt embroidered with a large sun on the shoulder, a reminder of our trip to the mountain top.

On another weekend, we went to a state park in Georgia with our friends, Tom and Becky. We rented a two-bedroom cabin near a waterfall in the park, and the four of us spent a special afternoon sitting on the bridge overlooking the water and enjoying each other in the sunshine. On the way home, we passed a newly opened McDonald's restaurant. Dare laughed and waved to Ronald McDonald in the parking lot. Right as she pointed, a van of young people drove by our car. The van door opened as they passed, and one of the occupants pulled his pants down and mooned us! I think Dare was so shocked to see this, but later we all laughed, wondering if Ronald McDonald was watching!

As we strolled along the lakeshore, the walkways were lined with the colors of different flowers. They were brilliant in the sunshine, and we would stop just to take a smell. At sunset, the mountain shadows reflected in the water. At nightfall, there was a cross shining from the hilltop, reminding us of His creation and its beauty. It truly was a place of serenity, with the awareness of God present as we developed a relationship of love. I would sleep on the floor next to her, listening to music by Andy Williams, Olivia Newton-John, and Roberta Flack.

There are so many stories to share of our time together during the fall of 1975 and early winter of 1976. But I was beginning to get both serious and confused in my thinking. I never imagined I would be so close to another person, nor did I think I would ever want to be in a long-term relationship for fear of marriage.

As we drew closer over the months, I also became increasingly frightened at the intimacy developing between us...a fear that made me question where we were headed in our future commitment. I didn't have a positive outlook on marriage, and questioned being with someone for the rest of my life. With these unsettling feelings growing, I decided to end our time together, and ran away from the commitment. Given the history of my childhood experiences with my parents' marriage, this became too scary.

Dare:

Our relationship had been wonderful. He was supposed to go home to meet my parents and siblings. we never had a major fight NOR disagreement. So I was heartbroken, confused, and sad when Keith broke up with me without a clear reason for his sudden decision to end the relationship. He said he wanted us to still "be friends."

I immediately took off the birthstone ring he had a jeweler design for me. When he gave it to me, he said it wasn't an engagement ring and if we were to ever breakup, he wanted me to keep it. Well, I wasn't in the mood to wear it and put it in the glove compartment of my car. I arranged to go to his apartment to bring my bicycle home. He wasn't there but left a note saying he wanted to remain close.

Keith truly broke my heart, but I wasn't going to chase

after him, and I wasn't going to take time to grieve for him. I'd spent nearly a year after breaking up with a former boyfriend, moping over the relationship. I was determined not to spend time like that ever again. I called everyone I knew to keep from calling him. I never intended to be fooled again by someone who could blindside me.

In May, I left Junaluska and returned to the campus of Western Carolina. I rented a trailer with a girlfriend by the Tuskegee river and attended summer school to obtain another certification in education. I started dating a student at Western who commuted from his home in Waynesville.

I heard Keith went to Canada with friends and was moving on with his life. I did buy a present for his 27th birthday. I left it at a friend's house and asked him to give it to Keith.

Keith:

I was depressed after my breakup with Dare, in deep thought about my fear of commitment and marriage. During my teenage years, I'd felt my mother's disappointment in her relationship with my father. She married him expecting him to enter law school, as had his father and four brothers. In fact, when she met my father, his dad was assistant attorney general for Presidents Roosevelt and Truman.

Granddad was a graduate of Harvard Law School, as were two of my dad's brothers. Dad's other two brothers received law degrees from Virginia University and Amherst Law School in Massachusetts.

Mom was a little spoiled, the middle child of three siblings and the only girl. Her father was a successful businessman and mother a registered nurse. She was her daddy's "little girl." Due to his business success, he was able to provide her with opportunities most girls weren't given during the depression years. For example, she grew up having her own bedroom and bath, music lessons, and social activities. In fact, one story she told was the time she took flying lessons in high school without her father's knowledge. She was successful in her academic studies, graduating from Furman University with a degree in education. Mom was a popular, attractive, Southern girl who was well dressed and steeped in social graces. Appearance and success were the most important values to her, and her parents' expectations were to find a man who would be as successful as her father...perhaps a doctor, a businessman, or an attorney.

When she met my father, she was attracted to his looks, personality, and plans to become an attorney. His mother and father, along with brother Paul, lived in a boarding home on Main Street Hendersonville. My father lived with his mother and younger brother while his father, my grandfather, was still active in government and living in Washington, D.C. Dad also had a history of asthma and his parents were told the climate in Hendersonville would be good for his health.

When my father met my mother, she worked in a camera-and-book store on Main Street Hendersonville. Both appeared interested in the other, and soon began to date. They attended Furman University together and continued dating on campus for a couple of years while in school. The courtship evolved and developed into a marriage proposal.

My father was Catholic and my mom was Baptist. She converted to Catholicism right before her marriage, as required by the Church. They were married on August 25, 1943 at the Church of The Immaculate Conception in my mom's hometown. There was a write-up of their marriage under the "The Woman's Page" section of the Hendersonville newspaper dated August 26, 1943. It not only described the ceremony and bridesmaids' gowns but included comments such as, "The elegant array of presents attested to the popularity of the young couple from prominent families." The article also stated, "The bride, widely loved for her vivacious and sweet charm of manner…," and described my father as, "…a young man held in high esteem, as well as being popular and accepted in law at Boston College, Boston."

This article gave the impression that mom must have had high dreams of success in marriage and in my father's completion of law school.

After the ceremony, Mom and Dad moved to Massachusetts, where my father attended Boston College Law School. My mother taught in the area, and within the year became pregnant with their first child. This was during World War II, and there was a shortage of medical doctors to provide adequate prenatal care. After the birth of my oldest brother, Mom became extremely ill with a kidney disease. When she told her parents of the illness, they persuaded her to return home to North Carolina. Her mother was a registered nurse and could provide daily care if Mom lived closer.

So, my father left law school and they returned to my mother's hometown. His plan was to return to Boston College Law School as soon as my mother was well.

However, this did not happen.

Given Dad's history of severe asthma he wasn't drafted into the war, but instead assigned to the wartime Chemical Corps of the U.S. Army. He commuted from Hendersonville to Morganton, North Carolina, which is an 80-mile drive one way. With their limited financial income, Mom's father helped them purchase a home located close to town. It had three bedrooms, a bath, a kitchen, a dining room, and living room. It also had a large yard, where I played with my siblings.

After the war, my father didn't return to law school, but accepted a position as an accountant at the local water department. He worked there for several years until his father-in-law helped him start a business selling and installing furnaces. This created additional stress in that Dad was not a businessman and would not collect the money owed to him after providing service. He lost money, creating financial issues in the marriage. My mother's father continued to assist in their financial relationship, bailing him out of difficulty. This eventually resulted in feelings of resentment toward Dad for not being able to provide for his family.

Since the Catholic church didn't believe in birth control, my mother ended up pregnant four times during the first nine years of marriage. In fairness to my mom, having children to rear in times of financial stress was hard. This was especially true when she still expected Dad to finish law school to become a successful attorney. While she tried to be a good, Catholic housewife and mother, her father felt she married beneath her social standing. I believe her parents added to the stress and financial pressure with their negative comments about having more children.

Dad decided to return to college to pursue a degree in teaching. I am not sure what happened to his dreams of completing law school, but it never happened. He graduated from Furman University, where he later received his master's degree. Mom taught school during these years to help with the financial stress. However, I think she preferred to be a housewife.

I remember feeling extreme stress during high school, hearing arguments between Mom and Dad because he wasn't as successful as anticipated and how she resented having four children due to the Church's doctrine. Angrily, she would say that she did not want "all these children," and if she had only listened to her father, she would have been "financially secure and living the life to which I was accustomed with my successful father."

Living in these years, I felt marriage was something I didn't want. Mom seemed very resentful of her social status, financial limitations, and responsibility for her children. I felt Dad's self-esteem was affected and his role as a strong husband and provider diminished. However, he remained very devoted to his family and committed to doing his best under the stress. His love was unconditional, his values strong.

I felt guilty, feeling I contributed to my mother's unhappiness and disappointment. I felt I wasn't really wanted, and worked extremely hard to gain her approval by behaving and doing household duties to ease the pressure and make her happy. I felt her love was conditional and that I had to be "perfect" to gain acceptance. I blamed myself for the stress in the family. I never thought it was anyone else's fault; it was me who was the problem. This observation affected my view of marriage and added to my fears of not being adequate as a husband.

In addition, when Mom enrolled me into boarding school during my ninth-grade year at Blue Ridge School for Boys, she had no idea what was going to happen. I grew up in a very sheltered and controlled home environment, and didn't feel adequate away from home. I was shy, depressed, and hurt by the move. It was during this upheaval that I was sexually abused by the headmaster of the school and an older roommate who was very manipulative. Being alone, confused, and scared, I participated in this affair. I called my father and told him that I was going to run away from this school if he didn't come to take me home.

I never told anyone of this abuse until I was an adult. This experience left me devastated and confused as an adolescent during my high school years. I was depressed and guilty that I hadn't been strong enough to stop the earlier abuse. I overcompensated by joining a multitude of high school activities. Some of these included being the president of the Distributive Education Clubs of America (DECA club), President of the PEP club, student council, Key club, newspaper staff, and winning the citizenship award my senior year. However, inwardly I continued feeling guilty, alone, and depressed. These outside activities were an attempt to convince myself that I was good. I never felt worthy nor felt others would accept me if they knew of the previous abuse.

The feelings regarding my parents' marital issues – along with the abuse that occurred while in boarding school – became a major block in committing to my relationship with Dare. I never told her of the reason for the breakup and needed time to sort through my issues.

We separated for four months. I had an opportunity to travel with friends to Canada, and during this trip I realized the strong connection we had in our relationship and didn't want to give up on the idea of marriage. I worked on my conflicts, gained confidence, and achieved a clearer idea of my goals. I realized I had made a huge mistake by running away and made the decision to repair what I had lost when I returned home. I learned Dare had completed her degree in education and accepted a teaching position in Asheville, North Carolina. She was also involved in dating another man.

On August 15, 1976, I left a note on her car window at her apartment asking to meet. She agreed and we began discussions. I stated that I wanted to date her again and, trying to redeem myself, explained the basis of my fears. I admitted there was a deeper meaning in our relationship that I didn't want to lose. Reluctantly, she agreed to try but wanted to take it slowly, saying she would date me while also continuing to see the other person. She was determined not to give up on that relationship if I wasn't committed to making ours work.

During the next few weeks, she was diagnosed with hives and I developed ulcerative colitis. We felt both the physical symptoms were a reaction to the stresses we faced. She took a weekend away to deal with answers to her concerns and I went under treatment for my colitis. Over the next month we continued to see each other and, with persistence, determination, and commitment, continued to work on our relationship.

Dare:

My childhood was happy and secure. We lived on 35 acres of property out in the country between Lilesville and Wadesboro, North Carolina. My mother was home with us until I was 15 years old. My dad had cows and gardened a lot, but was mostly a chicken farmer. I grew up primarily with my brothers and my little sister, Rebecca. I spent much of the time in my childhood trying to keep up with my brothers and prove I could do anything they could. They always said, "You can't do that because you're a girl!"

My parents met when Dad was 14 and Mom was 12. My dad grew up in Thomasville, North Carolina, right where there was electricity in town. He was the eighth child of 11 born to Jeannie Blake and Robert Lee Freeman. When Dad was 14, he, his parents, and three younger brothers moved to Anson County to live with his older, married sister and her husband.

My dad, being the oldest brother, tried to support the family due to his father's stroke and inability to work. Dad did not have an easy adolescent life, working nights while going to school during the daytime. He worked on a farm during the summer, plowing with a mule and receiving 50 cents a day and a sweet potato for lunch.

My mother was the oldest of seven children, five of them living. She was the only surviving girl until her mother had a little baby girl when Mom was 23 years old.

Neither of my parents had a lot of money, but they were both hard-working. They ended up graduating in the same class in 1942. My dad had dropped out after his dad died of a stroke. He moved to Washington, D.C. to live with an older brother and help deliver bread. He then returned to Anson County to finish high school. During their senior year, my parents gathered in the high school gym to listen to the president announce war. My mother said that most of the girls were crying and the boys looked somber. Dad was drafted and sent to Europe, where he was in the Battle of the Bulge and three other campaigns. He returned home after 37 months.

My mother was originally engaged to a soldier who was shot down over France and died. My parents met again in Wadesboro and dated for three years. Within a year of being married, they had my oldest brother, Richard. My mother was pregnant six times but lost the last baby. She said she wanted all of us and was heartbroken after the loss. She begged my dad to adopt, but he felt five children was enough!

I grew up in a small Methodist church with a membership of around 80 people. I had five generations of family members buried less than a mile from my home. My church family played a big part in my faith. My school talked about patriotism, good citizenship, and good character. We had prayer in school with devotions. The community met at our school for many events, and we were all remarkably close. I grew up with a family who valued its members and stressed the importance of life. While we knew we were all loved and wanted, we still had to toe the line! Our parents backed each other in discipline to keep us under control.

I was involved in the 4-H club and went to camp for several years. I was also involved in Future Teachers of America, Honor Society, and Future Homemakers of America. I was also a teenage bus driver the last two years of high school. I worked weekends at my uncle's store. My life was good.

While Keith and I had vastly different upbringings and experiences, I fell hard for him. My childhood was very secure, and I felt wanted by my parents, which is why I was so confused when we broke up. I didn't totally understand his experiences; I thought he had everything he could want. After all, my youth was filled with happiness and security.

Keith:

After I met with Dare in August of '76, I worked hard to repair our relationship and communication. In the middle of September 1976, I told her I wanted to marry. She replied, "When?" I said, "How about May of 1977?" Dare replied, "Ok, but I will continue to date the two of you until April."

I didn't like that answer and asked if she would consider an earlier time, perhaps during the Christmas holidays between our respective school breaks. I was afraid if I waited until May, she might decide to stay with her other relationship. Much to my delight, she agreed to an earlier wedding. We settled for December 18, 1976. And due to our engagement, she agreed to stop dating the other individual.

We met with the priest of the Catholic church to arrange the service. A favorite uncle of Dare's was in the Army, stationed in Turkey. He agreed to take his leave during that time so his wife could play the music for the ceremony.

Dare moved out of her one-bedroom apartment to a two-bedroom townhouse and began preparing for our home. The lease was up on my apartment in Hendersonville, and I moved into my parents' home until the wedding. Dare wanted a wedding in the mountains, and we agreed to the Catholic church where I had grown up. This created problems with my mother. She questioned why Dare wasn't marrying in her home church 200 miles away. However, Dare explained she had fallen in love with the mountains while in college the past four years. She also wanted her college friends to attend, and her campus minister to be part of the service.

This did not go well with either of our mothers. Dare's mom, who had returned to college after her children were grown, now felt Dare was moving too fast. She suggested waiting a year, saying she would have more time to help Dare with the planning if she could graduate first. In addition, I think she was concerned that Dare and I had discussed marriage too soon after getting back together. She felt a longer timeframe would provide more assurance the relationship would survive. But we didn't wish to wait and decided we wanted the ceremony to be in the western part of the state during the fall.

Dare wanted a small wedding. My mother wanted a large one so she could invite all relatives and friends from her town. We didn't send invitations since we were having a smaller gathering and decided not to register for wedding gifts. A formal wedding gown was put on layaway, but Dare later found another dress that appeared more appropriate for the service we desired. Therefore, the formal dress was rejected.

My mother had grown the wedding invitations to over 300, to which Dare was opposed. She feared walking down the aisle with so many people watching so she refused this number. She also felt overwhelmed with someone else planning and deciding things for her. Because tensions were high and disagreements were becoming more like arguments, we decided to move the wedding date again to avoid further disputes. We set the wedding date for October 16, 1976, which was the sweetest day on the calendar.

Several friends knew we had broken up for months and come back together planning a wedding! They also thought this was too fast but didn't know about the friction occurring with our parents.

However, we felt ready to celebrate life together and could deal with any problems that might arise.

Dare:

I knew I loved Keith with all my heart when we got back together. But I wasn't sure I trusted him and wondered if he just didn't like the idea of me dating someone else. I worried he might leave me again. Being with Keith was the main thing I wanted, and I wasn't terribly concerned about wedding plans. I wasn't interested in gifts because we had both lived on our own and had most of the needed household items. Also, I did not want others to be burdened with buying gifts. The only criteria I had for our wedding was I wanted a church wedding with God's blessing and a wreath in my hair. That was it!

I was incredibly happy about getting married. But I didn't know if he would show up at the church.

CHAPTER 2

THE WEDDING

Keith:

October 16, 1976 was a bright and sunny fall day. I woke that morning excited and looking forward to our wedding. I met Tom, a friend since high school, for breakfast and we discussed the activities of the day. First, I wanted to wash my car. Then I had to pick up the suit I was wearing for the night's celebration: a brown, vested, three-piece outfit that was especially tailored. The afternoon was spent with friends and family for last-minute preparations.

Our wedding ceremony took place at 7:30 p.m. It was a small gathering of 20 close friends and immediate family members. The Rev. George Weekley, a Methodist minister, and Father William Pharr, a Catholic priest, performed the service. Rev. Weekley was the campus minister at WCU and a friend to both of us. Father

Pharr was the Catholic priest at Immaculate Conception Church.

Dare chose words from *The Gift from the Sea* by Ann Lindbergh, significant because they reflected our feelings toward marriage and spoke of coming together as one while still being individuals. The church was decorated with yellow and white flowers. Dare nervously walked down the aisle with her father to the altar, where our vows were shared. Before we knew it, we were husband and wife.

Afterwards, we held a dinner reception at the Popular Lodge Inn in Hendersonville. To celebrate the occasion, my brother, Bill, and sister-in-law, Mary, made reservations earlier in the day for our wedding party. We laughed when cutting the wedding cake, not knowing there was cardboard between the layers. We kept pushing the knife blade through the cardboard until others in the crowd began to laugh and told us of the problem. We remained at the inn for several hours, visiting and talking. Soon Dare left with her mother to change into another outfit. Then we left for our motel.

I hadn't made early reservations for a honeymoon suite; I forgot about the fall tourist season with the changing colors of the trees, so there weren't any vacancies in a nicer hotel setting. The only vacancy in the area was an old, rundown motel. Certainly not what I envisioned for our first night together!

It was raining when we left the reception and arrived at the motel. We'd both had too much to drink, so we fell asleep in each other's arms. The following morning, we heard a lady yelling next door, "Clifford where are you?" Apparently, her dog had escaped the motel room. I looked at Dare and wondered what we got ourselves into. We left the motel rather early and went to breakfast at a local restaurant before visiting my parents. I think we were both glad to be away from that motel, and looking forward to moving into our new home and beginning our union!

Dare:

On the day of our wedding, I woke early and walked to the grocery store to buy food to prepare for the mid-day arrival of my parents and siblings. It was a gorgeous day – the sun was shining, fall leaves were in full color, and a gentle breeze was blowing. I went back to my apartment and cheerfully prepared a meal, excited and eagerly awaiting my family.

After the meal, I took my parents to meet Keith's parents. I was surprised to see Keith's mother in blue jeans. She later explained that she wanted them to feel comfortable, seeing that my family was from the country. I thought it was amusing because my mom wore more stylish clothing and never wore jeans. But it was nice of her to try and make my mom comfortable.

After the visit with Keith's parents, we came home to our apartment. My brother, Scott, and I sat on the couch eating tomato sandwiches and talking. My mom called from upstairs saying, "Dare, you need to hurry up and get dressed. I don't want these people to think I made you late. You would be late to your own funeral!" I had to argue back a bit because I was rarely ever late.

Soon we were all in the car, going to the church. When I learned that Keith really showed up, I suddenly became aware of what was going on and began to get nervous. While waiting for the service to start, I said to my dad, "I'm scared, is there a window I can jump out of?" My dad said, "It is going to be all right."

As the music started, my heart raced and I was

scared out of my mind. I held on to my daddy's arm as we headed down the aisle. As nervous as I got while walking down in front of only 20 family and friends, I don't think I could have made it in front of 300-plus people!

I settled down once I got beside Keith and in front of the minister and priest. The ceremony went well. We then went for the reception at Poplar Lodge where we ate dinner, cut the cake, and drank champagne.

I changed into another dress and we left for the motel. I was a little bit high from the alcohol when we arrived at the motel, and not exactly impressed with the accommodation. But I wasn't going to complain. I thought I had won the prize: this one-in-a-million man was my husband!

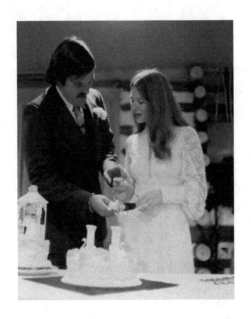

CHAPTER 3

MARRIED LIFE

Keith:

We rented our first home at Turtle Creek apartments in Skyland, a two-bedroom townhouse. The interior had an orange shag carpet which was the style at this time. We spent the weekend unpacking and settling into our home.

During one of our first weekends of marriage, we ventured out with neighbors on a camping trip to the Great Smokey Mountains National Park. This was our first-time attempt at camping. All seemed to be going well until the night, when we noticed a black bear coming through the campsite. It was looking for food and probably would not have bothered us. However, we quickly gathered up some survival equipment of blankets and food. I ran to the car while Dare went with the other lady to her van. We all spent the night in separate vehicles rather than sharing a tent. A great way to spend our first trip of married life!

One evening, back at our apartment, Dare was downstairs washing dishes and I was upstairs in our bedroom. I called to her through the air conditioning vent, saying, "Dare Freeman Ford, this is the Lord speaking." She answered, "What is it, Lord?" I continued, "You must be good to your husband!" She agreed and said, "I will, Lord!"

Well, a few nights later, she got back at me. She borrowed a pair of angel wings from a teacher friend. When I was asleep, she went to the closet and put on a white gown, a pair of wings, and a halo. She woke me up by saying, "Edmond Keith Ford, the Lord has sent me to tell you to be good to your wife!"

We always thought of tricks to play on each other during those first months of marriage. However, there were not always times of agreement. The adjustment to living together was hard when we had different expectations of our roles. For example, Dare constantly did everything for me: ironing, cooking, and greeting me with hugs and kisses when I came home from work. One afternoon I had to tell her to back off, that she was acting like a mother and smothering me. Of course, she responded by saying she wanted to be a good wife and thought this was the way to be. I responded, saying I had lived alone for over six years, was used to doing these things on my own, and didn't need her to do this for me. I said, "I married a wife, not a mother or a servant!"

Those are words I later came to regret, especially when I want some extra personal care!

Dare:

Adjustment to married life was much harder than I anticipated. When Keith told me I was smothering him, I didn't know how to act. I wanted to be a perfect wife, but suddenly the rules had changed. I thought I was loving, caring, and supportive. However, when Keith said he had been living by himself and taking care of his own needs, this changed my expectations of my role. The first week after marriage, while the wedding flowers were still sitting on the dining room table, I learned that my habit of chatting away was getting on his nerves. He said, "Dare, honey, I don't like to talk in the morning until I've had my shower and coffee." I'd been a morning person all my life and loved to get up talking!

The other adjustment was sharing a full-size bed; it was hard sharing at that size. I liked to sleep spread-eagle on my stomach. One of us generally ended on the floor by morning. Soon we had to purchase a queen-size mattress so we could both sleep comfortably.

One night I scorched the pan making popcorn and left it in the sink to soak overnight. When I came to bed, Keith was upset and had a stormy look. I asked what was wrong and he told me how angry he was that the pot was still in the sink. I was surprised by his reaction, but Keith has always been a perfectionist, never wanting a mess in his living environment. I should have known it when we were dating because he never wanted us to sit on his couch for fear of messing the cushions. He also never wanted to cook in the kitchen and preferred to eat out because he didn't want to dirty his dishes.

The popcorn pan was not the only thing I scorched; I accidently burned his dress shirt while ironing. Keith said, "Honey, I will iron my own shirts in the future." And I said, "That is fine with me." And he has!

We had both wonderful times and rocky times adjusting to married life! Thank goodness Keith changed over the years and I learned to iron better!

Keith:

We spent our first Christmas decorating a live tree with wooden ornaments that Dare had painted. We made love under that Christmas tree, a special memory of that holiday.

We remained at Turtle Creek until February 1977, when we moved to a house in Flat Rock, N.C. This house was owned by my uncle and was closer to my work. It also offered more room than the apartment. Although it wasn't closer for Dare's travel to school, she was near the interstate, which gave her better time.

Within the next month, I was surprised to receive a letter

from the graduate admissions office at the University of South Carolina in Columbia, where I had applied before meeting Dare. I had never completed the entire process, believing I wouldn't be accepted. However, the letter asked if I was still interested in graduate school. I thought that since they contacted me, my chances of acceptance might be good, so I continued the process.

Much to my delight and surprise, I was accepted. I convinced Dare to move to Columbia while I pursued a master's degree in clinical social work. With her certifications in five areas of education, I felt she could easily find a teaching appointment while I was a full-time student. She applied for and accepted a special education position in an elementary school in Columbia.

She began teaching in the fall of '77 and had a real adjustment to the environment. This was an inner city school in a predominantly black community, and the students were not only behind in their academic studies but came from home environments that were often disruptive. Dare tried to make a difference in each child's classroom experience, but had some difficulty with the behaviors displayed. Her style and interactions with these students soon settled into acceptance and love for them.

Dare:

I didn't know that Keith had applied to graduate school prior to our marriage, so I was surprised when I came home and Keith showed me the letter. I had started work on my masters at Western Carolina University, with night classes that met in Asheville. I had only taken a couple of classes when he presented the idea of moving to South Carolina. After discussion, I was okay with the move because I thought I could also further my education through the university in Columbia.

I held onto my position in Buncombe County until August. I was scheduled for surgery that month to remove a benign bone tumor on my left knee, which had created bursitis and caused pain when I moved my leg. I had the surgery, accepted the new teaching job by telephone, and began work in Columbia on crutches.

The school was in the middle of Columbia. I loved the students, but they were shocking to me. I learned their home lives were disruptive and their neighborhoods very rough; they knew so much about the struggles of the world. I was in a classroom trailer outside the main building, and the principal told me to come into the main building after the children left because it wasn't safe being in my classroom alone. I later learned from my mother, who read about it in a newspaper, that this principal was murdered a few years after we left Columbia.

There were 26 children from a children's home who attended Lyon Street Elementary school. Keith and I sponsored twin boys from the home on weekends and had them for a year until they returned to their mother. They were both challenging and rewarding for us.

I enjoyed Columbia. We lived in the Cliff apartments, on the ninth floor of married student housing. We had opportunities to attend activities, concerts, plays, and educational classes. We walked to the capitol building, saw President Ford and George McGovern, attended a concert with our favorite musician, John Denver, and Ms. America. We visited the Riverbank Zoo and spent our first anniversary at the state fair. It was an enjoyable adventure over the two years.

We had some issues regarding a close female friend of Keith's. I became threatened and very jealous. He tried to explain that this relationship was just someone he knew from his childhood. He had been a part of a support group during our separation and became close to her. I had never met her. Keith felt I was trying to control him, as his mother had controlled his father, and was determined not to let this happen. I felt that he was too emotionally attached in this relationship. I wanted to be the "perfect" wife and could not understand why he would be so close to this lady. We had many arguments and were both too stubborn to give in.

In reality, we were fighting over issues that had nothing to do with this relationship. Because of earlier comments from friends who questioned our decision to marry, we weren't going to let this issue lead us to separation. Luckily, after many hurt feelings, we resolved the real issues underneath the confusion and the communication greatly improved.

Keith:

During the first year of graduate studies I spent so much time writing papers that I thought I would turn into a typewriter. At one point, the stress hit hard, and I considered dropping out of school. However, Dare was always there to support and encourage me to continue.

With commitment, hard work, and her support, I was successful in my studies and ended with honors.

After graduation, we weren't sure if we would remain in Columbia or return to the mountains of North Carolina. Until that decision was made, I took a position as an assistant apartment manager at the Dargan apartments in Columbia. However, we longed for the mountains of North Carolina and decided to move back. Dare was offered a position teaching in the Buncombe system where she had previously worked. I began searching for employment in my field of social work.

After several months of searching, I was hired as a clinical social worker in the adolescent unit at Highland Hospital, an inpatient psychiatric facility owned by Duke University. We rented a small, two-story house in Woodfin from an elderly woman named Ruth Wilcox, who was retired and had several small houses and trailers on her property. Dare and I were incredibly happy to be back in the mountains, with our own little home and good jobs.

When we moved into the house, our landlady was clear that she didn't rent to couples with children or pets. But when I received my first paycheck Dare said, "Let's have a baby." I replied, "Dare, honey, we have no money saved and we cannot afford a baby. We've just started new jobs."

Dare replied, "We can start saving now. If one of us is sterile, then we will adopt. Remember all the x-rays you had for colitis? I might be sterile myself! I read in a magazine that it takes a married couple an average of eight months to become pregnant, so that's seventeen months before a baby is even here."

However, within the month, when we were visiting Dare's parents during the Christmas weekend, Dare told her aunt how tired she was and that she had difficulty buttoning an outfit she was going to wear to church on Christmas. She continued by saying that she had swollen lymph nodes under her armpits and her gold rings were turning her finger black.

Her aunt, who worked for a physician, stated, "Dare, you may be pregnant," and suggested that we send a urine sample to the doctor's office in the morning for a pregnancy test. The next afternoon, on December 24th, Aunt Bonnie called to say, "Congratulations! Start dancing, you're going to be parents!" We were shocked but happy.

That same night, we went to Dare's grandmother's house for a family Christmas party. When leaving the party, Dare slipped on wet steps and fell. I was so upset, saying, "Is the baby ok?" She laughed and said, "This baby is no bigger than a pea and we are both just fine."

Upon returning home after that weekend, we were afraid to tell our landlady, thinking she would make us move. However, she was delighted and welcomed our new addition.

Dare:

The next few months we prepared for our baby. It was an exciting time as we anticipated the birth of our child. However, the summer was extremely hot, and I was uncomfortable without air conditioning in the house. Keith purchased a window conditioner for comfort, and I mostly stayed upstairs in our bedroom, trying to stay cool.

My pregnancy went well overall. One Sunday afternoon in January we took a long ride. I noticed some light bleeding, and it scared both of us, thinking we might lose the baby. The bleeding stopped and we decided not to take any longer rides for a while.

The doctor said he usually only allowed 20 pounds of weight gain during pregnancy, but because I was so thin, he allowed me to gain 25 pounds. Halfway through the pregnancy I was placed on a restrictive diet because he thought I was gaining too much, too fast. He said I could have JELL-O for dessert and one tablespoon of mashed potato for a meal. He didn't want me to struggle to take weight off after the birth. I only gained 25 pounds and felt good until the delivery.

Elizabeth Dare Freeman Ford was born August 19, 1980 at Pardee Hospital in Hendersonville, N.C. The doctor induced labor around twelve thirty, and Elizabeth was born three hours and forty minutes from the first pain. I knew I was lucky not to have a long labor for the first baby.

I was given a saddle block (called caudal anesthesia) to numb me before being placed on the delivery table. The spinal fluid leaked, giving me an excruciating headache that would last for ten days. No medication took care of the pain. I felt like an axe was splitting my head open. When I returned home, the headache continued.

To give me a break, Keith took Elizabeth for a car ride, placing her across his lap. He took her to the mall where he walked her. She was five days old the first time he did this outing. Keith said he wasn't comfortable having my mom come to stay with us; he wanted to take care of us himself. Several friends brought us meals.

We had a lot to learn about parenting. We never put Elizabeth down for fear she would cry. For three days and nights, Keith and I took turns holding her until we were exhausted and had to put her down in the bassinet. She cried for about three minutes and went fast to sleep.

I was able to stay home with Elizabeth that year, which was one of the best times of my life. I spent time dressing her in different outfits and taking lots of pictures.

Because one of my cousins lost a child to SIDS (sudden infant death syndrome), I constantly checked on Elizabeth through the night and during her naps. When she was five months old, she was hospitalized due to complications from croup and bronchiolitis. She was in respiratory distress and placed in an oxygen tent.

They wanted to put a bronchial dilator in to help her breathing before taking x-rays. That night, Keith's parents offered to stay with her until we could go for supper. When we returned to the room, I noticed there was no mist in the tent. I went to the nursing station and discovered they had forgotten to add the medication. When I told the physician the next morning, he was furious and had discussions with the nursing supervisor. The next morning one of the male nurses said he was so relieved that she was better because he worried about her condition when he left the previous night.

They had Elizabeth in the same room with a baby who had the flu. I asked the doctor if we could discharge her and take her to Keith's parents' home. Seeing that they lived near the hospital, he discharged her and we took her to Keith's parents' home. We are so thankful that she recovered.

Being a new mother was wonderful, but I became concerned with every fever, cough, or earache. She once choked on a cracker at nine months. Fortunately, I had read on how to do the Heimlich maneuver and was able to loosen the cracker out of her throat. It flew about five or six feet across the room. I was so grateful that she was okay.

Keith:

We wanted a bigger house, and in the summer of 1981 found one in a subdivision known as Bent Creek, in the western part of Asheville. We rented with an option to buy within the year. This was a brick split-level house, a popular home style, with three bedrooms, two bathrooms, a den, a living room, a kitchen, and a deck. Life was settled and good.

We loved our new home. The neighborhood offered wide roads, where we spent afternoons walking with Elizabeth in her stroller. She loved it when we approached a hill and I let the stroller go. It would pick up speed down the hill and I would run beside her as she laughed with excitement. Of course, Dare would be yelling, "Stay with her, she might fall out or a car might be coming!" I didn't pay much attention to these concerns. I knew she was safe, and I would be able to catch her if needed. Later, I was able to put a carrier on the back of my bicycle and take her for rides around the neighborhood. She loved the breeze and would squeal with delight.

Shortly after this move, we found a small Methodist church we loved not far from home. One Sunday afternoon, I took Elizabeth alone to this church while Dare was home working on schoolwork. Several members of the congregation were very welcoming and paid attention to Elizabeth. I met the minister, who welcomed us to the area. Upon checking out the church and returning home, I felt comfortable and told Dare that I wanted us to go back the following week.

I was extremely impressed when the minister welcomed us back and called me by name! Our family continued to attend this church and I participated in services and Sunday school classes. We made several friends and socialized with them by having their company in our home.

In 1983 my work at Highland Hospital needed further growth, challenge, and experience. I interviewed for a new position as a program manager and clinical social worker at Appalachian Hall, another inpatient psychiatric hospital in Asheville. This position gave me social work and administrative experience in addition to a salary increase in my duties as program director of the new adolescent unit.

Dare and I were happily involved in church, jobs, and community activities. We discussed having another child (on the telephone!) while she was visiting her parents. When she returned home, we began The Baby Project. In July of 1983, we learned we were pregnant again. We were excited to have another child as part of our family. We weren't sure of the sex.

Dare:

My second pregnancy didn't go as well as the first. When I passed a huge slab of what looked like raw calf liver the size of the palm of my hand, I thought I was losing the baby. It was a blood clot, and when I consulted with my OB/GYN physician, he said he didn't think I had lost the baby yet. He couldn't promise that I would keep it. I asked if there was anything I could do to prevent it, and he said, "There are no promises, but if you want to go to bed, keep your feet elevated, and rest, that is about all you can do." So I did that very thing and spent the entire Labor Day weekend in bed with my feet up, praying all the time.

I felt more relaxed once I hit the end of the first trimester. Then I went to the OB/GYN for my next appointment. The technician doing the ultrasound said there were developmental concerns because the head measured smaller than the rest of the body. The recommendation was to eat lots of protein and come back in three weeks for a repeat of the ultrasound. While waiting in the hallway to speak with the doctor, I told Keith, "Oh no! The baby might be a microcephalic baby." When the doctor spoke with us, he told us to eat protein, "think happy thoughts," and return in three weeks. I said, "Hmm, that was interesting. I'm supposed to think happy thoughts?"

Three weeks later, we returned for the repeat ultrasound. This time we couldn't believe our ears when they told us the baby's head was now too big, out of proportion to the rest of its body. Again, Keith and I were in the hallway waiting to speak with the doctor. I said, "Oh my gosh, now we are talking about a hydrocephalic baby." I worried the baby might need a shunt to take off pressure from the fluid. When the doctor came to speak with us, he said, "Come back in December. Just go home and think happy thoughts," as if happy thoughts would make everything better.

In December, Keith wasn't able to make the appointment, so I went alone. We had invited a dozen people from our Sunday School class to our house that night, and I felt in a rush to get home to get ready for the company. The news I got that day: "Now the baby seems to have the right proportions, but I must tell you the baby is breech." I asked about the breech and was told the doctor may be able to turn the baby; if not, I would need a cesarean section.

I cried all the way home. When Keith saw me, he looked concerned and asked, "Dare, what's wrong? Is the baby okay?" I told him that I might have to have a C-section and that I would look like World War III. Keith hugged me and said, "I would love you even if you looked like a nuclear war." We ended up cancelling our commitment that night due to being too stressed to have company.

When I returned to the doctor at the end of January, I was told the baby was no longer breech and now in the right position. However, my blood pressure was too high and I needed to get it under control, or they were going to have to admit me to the hospital. I spent the rest of the pregnancy trying to keep my feet elevated.

The baby was due March 17, but on March 10 we all went to the circus. While there, I started the beginning phase of labor with a cramp on my right side. In the early morning hours, I woke and told Keith I was in labor; my contractions were close. I took a bath and put on my makeup. Keith woke Elizabeth and dressed her. We left her with our minister's wife while we went to the hospital.

Everything was going as expected but the epidural did not take in my right leg. I asked for more medication and the nurse rolled her eyes as if I were faking and wanted medication. I was so upset and wanted to smack her. She would say, "You won't get any more medicine until you get off the gurney and up on the table." I was in such pain and couldn't get up. I continued to bite on a washcloth in my mouth to take the pressure off my body. A student nurse was in the room who wanted to sit by me to watch the birth. She was so irritating as she just sat there, shaking her leg right beside me. I was stressed but didn't tell her to stop. This was the last opportunity she had to observe while in school, but it was distracting to me.

I was rolled into the delivery room and Andrew Robert Keith Ford was born on March 11, 1984 at 9:11 am on a Sunday morning. He weighed seven pounds, 10.5 ounces and had a head full of blond hair. The nurse placed him on my chest, and once again, I was in love with my child. I was incredibly happy and relieved he was healthy.

Keith called his father and told him of the news. His father broke down and cried when Keith told him we had named the baby Robert, after him. We left the hospital for home when he was 30 hours old because we had to wait until he was circumcised. Keith buckled him in the new car seat for the 30-minute ride home.

Despite all the stress of my pregnancy with Andrew, when I looked at him I felt it was all worth it.

When he was three weeks old, he was exposed to chickenpox. He didn't contract the virus, but his sister, Elizabeth, was covered. Andrew seemed to settle in during the next few months. I returned to work when he was two months old. He was placed in a private home, but the lady became pregnant again and could no longer keep him. Our church opened a daycare center, and we entered Andrew in October of 1984. The director of the center was a very warm and caring provider by the name of Mary. She was excited, having just opened the program, and Andrew became the first and only baby enrolled in the infant room. He got a lot of attention from the adults and older children in the program.

Three weeks after the daycare opened, Andrew woke after a Sunday afternoon nap at home. I gave him a bottle in the playpen in the kitchen while I cooked lunch. I then put him in his crib for a nap. We had plans to visit another couple from our church that afternoon, and when I went to wake him up, Andrew had a fever. I called our friends to cancel the visit, but the lady insisted that they were not afraid of Andrew's fever and to come over to their house. We went to visit but while we were there, Andrew became extremely sick and vomited. We took him to the urgent care center, where he received a diagnosis of an ear infection. They gave him antibiotics and we took him home.

Later that night his fever was higher, and he didn't seem like himself. By the next morning, he didn't appear to feel any better. His coloring was greyish, and he looked lethargic. I stayed home from school and called the pediatric office. A receptionist said, "I wouldn't be too concerned. You know it can take up to 72 hours for antibiotics to work."

I said, "Well, he is not acting like himself. I would really like him seen." She sounded somewhat irritated and said, "Well, if it will make you feel better, you can bring him in...but not till 3:00." I told her I would be there.

When I got into the office, the pediatrician saw him and a lady from the office drove us immediately to the pediatric intensive care unit (PICU) at the hospital. The staff started tests to evaluate the situation. I called Keith to inform him of the event, and he came directly to the hospital. I stayed with Andrew throughout the night. They confirmed a diagnosis of Spinal Meningitis B.

He was hospitalized for four days in the PICU and an additional ten days on the pediatric ward. There were concerns as to whether or not he would survive. Also, there were possible future problems with learning disabilities, deafness, blindness, hyperactive disorder, and problems walking. While in PICU, his coloring looked very grey. I prayed to God, saying, "God, he was yours before he was mine. I give him back to you if that is your will. Just help me to help Keith and Elizabeth get through this." After this prayer, I felt total peace overcome my body. I looked up and my baby's coloring turned from grey to rosy. I knew people might think I was crazy, but I know a miracle happened before me.

Some of his treatments while in the hospital were concerning for their side effects, but we felt there was no choice in order to give him the best chance for recovery. While in the hospital, he received physical therapy to lean how to crawl again and eat solid food. After his tenth day in the ward, he was much better and discharged home. Both Keith and I watched him closely for several months for other difficulties.

Andrew kept getting high fevers over the next few months because his immune system had been weakened. At eleven months, Andrew was back in the hospital for a fever. The doctor didn't want to take any chances, so Andrew spent three days there. In addition to all the stress of sickness and worry, he had two sets of ear tubes placed, one of which became embedded and had to be removed surgically.

With ear infections with both kids, we were busy at the urgent care center. Many friends laughed and said, "You guys have paid for that building." Regardless of the illnesses, I've never regretted being a mom and loved my children with all my heart. I always wanted to be a mother and even looked forward to being a grandmother. Family was the most important value to me.

Keith:

When I first heard of the second pregnancy, I knew exactly when it happened. Dare had been out of town visiting with her parents, and when she returned home, she brought our nephews to visit. Our daughter was excited to have her cousins staying with us. They were all active and entertained each other.

After the kids were in bed, Dare and I had a romantic interlude on our upper deck off the kitchen. One of these nights was my birthday. When she told me she was pregnant, I couldn't help but think he was conceived on my day. I thought it was a great way to celebrate my special day! We sometimes refer to him as our "deck baby."

The next nine months were stressful with the pregnancy. On the day of his delivery, I was surprised and excited to have a son. I was delighted to have both a daughter and a son.

Over the first months, Andrew did well. There were no major difficulties. However, the day before his hospitalization for the spinal meningitis, he had an ear infection and that is how the physician felt he ended up with the virus. During the time of Andrew's sickness, I commuted back and forth from home to the hospital, taking care of Elizabeth while Dare was with Andrew. I worried about his survival during the first few days of his hospitalization in the PICU. Every time the phone rang at home, I was scared to answer for fear of hearing about his death. I was absolutely amazed at Dare's response to the situation. Night after night she remained at his side, overseeing his condition and providing love. I was worried about her health, too. She wouldn't leave his room, didn't sleep well, and refused to go home for the two weeks of his stay.

I remember the doctor telling her that she needed to rest and return home for a night. She kept telling Dare they would call our home if his condition changed. Finally, one night after being up for several hours by his bedside, I was able to convince her to come home for a good night's sleep. However, she wasn't comfortable, thinking and worrying about his status. She finally told me that she didn't care if she was sleeping or not, she was staying at the hospital to be by her baby. There was no convincing her otherwise. She returned the next morning and stayed until he was finally discharged.

I learned a lot about a mother's love as I watched Dare's interaction and concern for his wellness. At times when

I was exhausted and overwhelmed from the stress of his illness, caring for Eliza and maintaining my work schedule, Dare pushed in with Andrew. I know how much she loves her children and will neglect her own needs to attend to her child. Dare always wanted to be a mother. To her, this has been the most important gift given. Watching her in this situation gave me an appreciation for maternal love.

I was so grateful when he was discharged home. Whatever developmental problems he faced, I knew we would do this together and accept the consequences. Because of his diagnosis, there were 45 people exposed in the daycare center who had to have medication to prevent the illness.

CHAPTER 4

JACKSONVILLE

Keith:

One afternoon in the fall of 1985, I received a telephone call from a representative of Brynn Marr Hospital in Jacksonville, North Carolina. She was recruiting for a program director of their children and adolescent unit. I gave her the name of several people who might be interested in the job. While on the phone, she asked if I would be interested in interviewing. I stated I wasn't seeking a change of position. However, since I planned to be in that area for a conference the next week, she asked if I would be willing to meet with her. I agreed to stop by and explore the situation.

I flew to Jacksonville, and the assistant administrator of the hospital met me at the airport. We drove to the hospital and toured the facility. The unit I would be responsible for had a 20-bed adolescent/10-bed children's program.

The ward needed some renovations completed due to destruction caused by unruly patients.

I was concerned by what I saw. I questioned the criteria for referrals they accepted and whether adequate supervision was provided in the environment. I was told that the entire program needed restructuring. They hoped the new manager could provide solutions. Having had previous experience with program design, I felt confident this could be accomplished. In the past, I had implemented several management programs similar to what I felt Brynn Marr sought.

After touring the hospital, the assistant administrator and unit manager took me on a tour of the town. We drove by Camp Lejeune, a well-known military base for the U.S. Marine Corps. We then drove to Emerald Isle, which was 25 miles from the hospital. I was struck by the sights and sounds of the area. I heard seagulls and rolling waves, and saw many summer homes. I've always loved the beach, with its warm weather and relaxing environment.

After my visit to Jacksonville and the surrounding area, I was impressed enough to agree to an interview with corporate representatives and other medical staff. Arrangements were made for Dare to fly back with me to Jacksonville within two weeks.

When I returned home and talked with Dare, she was surprised and somewhat reluctant to think about giving up all we had in our current lives. I explained that I thought it would be a good career advancement and a salary increase. I described how nice it would be living close to the beach. Dare agreed to fly with me to check it out. We arranged time off and flew to explore the opportunity. We were both open to a possible move, but not yet ready to commit. There were still unanswered questions as to housing, a job for Dare, daycare concerns, and schools for Elizabeth. While Dare agreed to explore the area, she wanted the opportunity to learn more about employment possibilities with the school system.

During my meeting with representatives, I quoted a salary $10,000 more than my current income. I felt that I had nothing to lose and didn't expect them to agree. For some unknown reason, they accepted my request, and agreed to pay for moving costs, assist in housing relocation, and help Dare locate a teaching position. It felt like too generous an offer to refuse. After discussing with Dare, we were both on board with the offer and pursued the opportunity.

While in Jacksonville, someone in the hospital told me of a house that was for rent by a Marine captain and wife who were looking for tenants due to a transfer. We met with the wife and arranged a tour of the home. I was excited to find the house was in a nice subdivision named Stillwood. The neighborhood looked exceptionally clean and the lawns very well kept.

Dare was also perfectly fine with renting the house; we had a place to live. Dare interviewed with Onslow County schools. Being a military town, there were always openings. She was offered a job at Blue Creek Elementary school, about four miles from the home we had just rented.

We returned to Asheville and started preparing for the move. We turned in our resignations and began telling friends, family, and coworkers good-bye. While this sudden and out-of-the-blue decision appeared crazy to some, we both felt it was worth the challenge. We placed our house on the market and sold it within three weeks. We were happy, even though we lost money on the transaction. We didn't want to maintain a home in the mountains along with one on the coast, and didn't know whether or not we would return to the mountains. We wanted to put our focus on one home and community at the time.

We moved the first part of November in 1985. The Stillwood house had three bedrooms, two baths, a kitchen, and a living room, and was within five miles of the hospital. The house was perfect for our family and convenient for our jobs.

Coming into the school system in November, the principal allowed each teacher to give Dare three students of their choice to set up her new class. So you can imagine what kind of a classroom she received! Therefore, Dare got another challenge!

Once I started my new job, I learned the hospital had a terrible reputation in the community. I had the task of working to improve this relationship. The previous manager had been unable to control the outburst in adolescent behavior issues. So we revised the criteria for admission to curtail the number of court-referred delinquent patients with criminal records. We also developed a management program to address destructive violence, with closer supervision of behavioral outbursts. Staff members attended workshops designed to improve communication skills for working with adolescents. A point system for awards and privileges was implemented for the patients. Group therapy centered on accountability for behaviors. We worked hard to improve and increase the census, and slowly accomplished our objectives.

Living in Jacksonville gave me a great sense of freedom; I had never lived in another place that offered a sense of making it on my own without family nearby. Having Dare at my side was the support and encouragement I needed to make a name for myself. I wasn't just my parents' child, nor did I feel that community people were watching to make sure I lived up to the standards my mom expected of me. I bought a new T-top convertible and rode to the beach feeling independent and free. I even rode at times with my shirt off to gain the suntan I wanted. My mother would have never allowed this around our hometown. Afterall, what would the neighbors think?

Dare and I had our two children and a sense we could make our own decisions without approval from other family members. Again, this was one of the advantages of living farther away and close to the beach, which I loved. However, Dare wasn't happy living in this predominantly military town, nor in her teaching position; she didn't want to rear our children in this environment. Life in Jacksonville was settling down, but our emotional ties were still attached to the mountains of western North Carolina. We knew Jacksonville would not be a permanent living arrangement.

Dare:

When Keith first talked of moving to Jacksonville, my left upper arm started tingling vigorously. I squeezed it tightly between my fingers and the thumb on my right hand, which made the tingling stop. I had so much running through my mind. I was happy in our neighborhood, our church, and my job. Life started rushing quickly as we prepared to take the leap of faith.

The hospital flew us down. We rented a car from the airport and drove to the town. I could not believe how flat and straight the roads were. I hadn't been in the flatlands in quite a while. I began feeling the excitement of getting ready for a big adventure.

The next morning, I interviewed with the Onslow County administration. This meeting went well and, before I knew it, I was offered a job at Blue Creek Elementary school teaching language arts and reading to fourth, fifth, and sixth grade regular students. Keith's interview at the hospital was fine. He was offered the position and told we had three weeks to move.

Soon our little family of four was packed and ready

for the seven-and-a-half-hour drive to the coast. Keith drove his blue Honda Civic and I had a brown Chevette. Neither car was big enough to carry much. Keith had a broom and mop hanging out his window. I had the kids, and the job of trying to entertain them for the journey. I followed Keith and felt we looked like vagabonds headed for the promised land!

We arrived before our furniture was delivered and slept on the living room floor in an empty house without knowing anyone. That night the doorbell rang. Keith sauntered to the front door, and when he cautiously opened it encountered our first guest. It was the minister from Northwood Methodist Church who welcomed us to Jacksonville. We didn't know how he knew we were there. We guess he got our name from either the hospital or school system. The next day, the moving van arrived, and we were busy unpacking boxes.

Life began to settle during the next few months. My teaching job was a challenge the first year, but I tried to make the best of the situation. Near the end of this year, I seriously considered leaving the teaching profession to obtain a real estate license. However, I decided that wouldn't be a good move for my family. I would be called away to show houses day and night, and weekends. I didn't want to leave them.

My second and third years went much more smoothly than the first. In fact, in one delightful year I had two-thirds of my students who were motivated and highly functional. The other third needed extra help. I grouped the children in such a manner that they all worked helping each other.

One of the first encounters we had in Jacksonville was fire ants in the front yard. Elizabeth was bitten by several as she leaned on a tree while waiting for Andrew and me to drive to school. One of my coworkers said, "Oh yes, Jacksonville is full of them. It's very painful when they bite." A few months later, Andrew, at only 20 months of age, managed to get into a bed of fire ants on the edge of the backyard deck. They crawled up the pant legs on his coveralls. This was an experience we hadn't experienced in the mountains.

The owners of the Stillwood home decided to put the house on the market. We weren't ready to buy a home there, so we moved to an older subdivision right behind Stillwood, into a Cape Cod-style house on Diane Drive with a large, fenced-in backyard. It had a small kitchen, a dining room, a living room, one bedroom and bath downstairs, and three bedrooms and one bath upstairs. The floors were all hardwood. While we liked the house, we didn't like the water bugs that came out at night on the side of the house. We believe that the enormous number of water bugs were due to a nearby drainage ditch which enticed them. Therefore, we made the decision to move again.

Our third and final home was our favorite. It was in an area closer to town, near Jacksonville High School. We thought we would escape all the water bugs crawling on the side of the house at night if we moved to a nicer area. The home had many benefits. It had four large bedrooms and two full bathrooms upstairs. Downstairs it had a living room, a dining room, a bedroom, a full bath, an eat-in kitchen, a laundry room, and a den with a fireplace. There was also a fenced-in backyard. I really loved that house.

Keith kept taking me around to look at houses to buy. But I didn't want to rear my daughter in a military town with young Marines running around. As Elizabeth grew to adolescence, I didn't want her around a "jungle" of men who might distract her from a formal education. The heat and humidity in Jacksonville were also such that in the summer my lungs would ache. I didn't know if we would ever go back to the mountains, but I wasn't in favor of investing in a permanent home.

There were many fun and enjoyable things to see and do in Jacksonville, and outings that involved adventure. The time spent in the area added special memories and experiences to our reasons for making the move. I discovered the many pawn shops, which were exciting to visit because I never knew what I would find and it was always enjoyable to see what would be new. I specifically would look for deals with jewelry. I found many good pieces including rings, bracelets, and earrings, including a large citrine, blue topaz, and an onyx ring for Keith. I purchased a Ronnie Millsap tape that I played on my way to and from work. Elizabeth finally told me, "Mom, I'm sick of hearing that music."

Our family loved going to Topsail Beach and Emerald Isle on weekends, both fun towns to visit. Several people told us we would love living at the beach. I said, "Not while we have little children with constant ear infections and needing medical facilities at night." I didn't want to drive 45 miles to get medical attention. On occasion, Keith and I hired a babysitter so we could have a night out. However, by the time we paid the babysitter and bought dinner, snacks, and several movies for them, we barely had enough money to eat at a McDonald's. Regardless, I just enjoyed sharing an evening out with Keith.

One weekend we took the children to Fort Macon, where we picnicked and toured the fort. Both the children enjoyed history and liked it when we traveled to various museums and art centers. Another trip was to New Bern, where we visited Tryon Palace, the state capital before it was moved to Raleigh. Elizabeth spent several hours touring the home and artifacts.

We met and would visit several good friends. I remember when Keith and I needed outfits for a costume party and found a man who rented costumes. It looked like a lot of fun. From that visit, I kept the thought in my head as a possible business idea for future reference. We also went to several other parties organized by the hospital. I loved dancing with Keith, and one of our favorite songs was "Lady Dressed in Red."

I also liked Andrew's daycare, and loved his daycare teacher, Ms. Terry. She had a bird named Teapot that Andrew would talk about all the time.

During my time in Onslow County, my health was good. I joined Weight Watchers® and obtained my lifetime membership. I lost enough weight that my eyes became hollow, my cheek bones poked out, and I looked like a skeleton with a big smile. I thought I looked so good but Keith said, "Dare, you need a little more meat on your bones."

Besides ear infections, Andrew fell and cut his forehead while dancing in daycare. I was in the process of baking a cake for Elizabeth's sixth birthday when I got the call. I had to stop and take him to urgent care, so I never got the cake done and had to buy a store cake. Another time, Andrew fell at daycare and cut his tongue all the way through. Another trip to urgent care! The doctor said it was a bad cut, but he didn't feel the need for stitches because tongues heal naturally.

The only other little health incident with Andrew was when he had a "startle reflex" while swinging on the playground. We were told we should take him to a neurologist, thinking he had a seizure. Due to his history of spinal meningitis, we felt more comfortable traveling back to Asheville. He was evaluated and it was concluded that he did not have a seizure and was fine. But the reflex scared the workers at the daycare.

Elizabeth's health was good except for complaining of chest pains one time while we were at a restaurant. She grabbed her chest and cried due to the pain, so I left Keith with Andrew and escorted her to the doctor. The doctor felt she was fine but may have had reflux from her meal. He also made a comment that she was quite dramatic and made a "big racket" while experiencing her pain.

Keith had a flare-up of his colitis. It concerned me that he seemed so tired and anemic because of the blood loss. I wondered if it would ever get better. I was running three and four times a week to the pharmacy to get his medicine. One night Keith had severe pain that radiated from his back around to his stomach. I dropped the kids off with a friend and drove him to Onslow Hospital. It was a dark and rainy evening as we drove down the road. He said he was going to throw up, so I quickly pulled off the side. When we arrived at the ER, it seemed forever before the paperwork was completed for admission. He was squirming in pain and miserable; I was afraid he might die right in front of me.

After evaluation, Keith was admitted to the hospital with a kidney stone which, after two days did not pass. On the third day, Keith called to say that the doctor wanted to transfer him to another hospital so they could do a procedure to break up the stone. I was writing reports and had to decide whether or not to be out of the classroom for a few days. I contacted a friend to take the kids while I was gone. This happened to be the day Elizabeth watched the space shuttle, which exploded after liftoff.

I was soon driving him to Fayetteville for admission to Highsmith–Rainey Hospital. Our experience was a good one and everything went according to expectation. Keith was a goofball when he returned to the room after his procedure. I ordered a special gourmet steak meal complete with flowers, white tablecloth, and wine. I wanted us to celebrate. Since neither of us wanted the wine, I took it to a coworker who was also at the hospital for his wife. Keith was discharged the next morning.

CHAPTER 5

BACK TO THE
MOUNTAINS

Keith:

Oddly enough, my father called one evening to relay
that the local hospital in Hendersonville was opening
a new adult psychiatric inpatient unit. Having the ideal
experience, I made the decision to apply. This unit
consisted of a contract between Pardee Hospital and
Mental Health Management out of Washington, D.C. The
management company supplied the administrative staff
and medical support team while the hospital provided
the space, nursing staff, and administrative support. I
would be employed by the management company for the
position of program director. I submitted the application
and was offered the position. The move occurred in the
summer of 1988.

I was involved with the design and construction plans for the unit in addition to writing policy and procedures, hiring staff, and orienting medical staff to the new psychiatric service. The unit opened in July of 1988. The following month we had our first state inspection, which went well.

Being a new service for the hospital and the community, many medical providers were reluctant to place patients in a locked facility. We needed to educate them so they understood the value of sending patients to a community program vs. a state-run facility two hours away. Medical providers changed their minds, however, when the first patient admitted was a 69-year-old lady experiencing severe memory loss, depression, and confusion. After medical and psychiatric evaluation, we discovered she suffered from a brain tumor which caused interruptions to her mental health. She was transferred for surgery and recovered. Her referring physician was surprised and delighted that we discovered the problem.

We had an exceptionally good team of professional clinicians and nursing staff to make the program successful. But the responsibility of building the census was too much of a strain and conflict for me. Working for a management company based in Washington, D.C. while dealing with local hospital administration became unbearable. I received daily telephone calls from the management company harassing me about the census, marketing plans, and what I was doing to increase referrals. Although I was marketing with various community referral agencies and medical staff, I just couldn't round up enough people to be admitted.

I began to see my health affected; I wasn't able to sleep and had heart palpitations, chest pains, and depression. Still, I remained in the position for four years before deciding it wasn't worth the physical problems I experienced. I decided to resign.

I then took a position with two psychiatrists at their agency, known as Center for Change. I was a clinical social worker counselling outpatient clients and helping as the office manager. I began work there in 1992, and it was during this time that my wife and I began a new chapter in our lives.

Dare:

I was so happy returning to the mountains from Jacksonville, and glad to be back in the Buncombe County school system. I was assigned to a middle school with my former boss, who had been transferred to North Buncombe Middle School. He had been my principal at Erwin Middle School in West Asheville. I was also excited to be home again with former friends and coworkers. While the move to Jacksonville was an interesting time, I felt so comfortable returning to Western North Carolina. I had to drive further to school but it was an enjoyable ride, looking at the mountains and feeling the change in weather.

We initially moved into an apartment for three weeks before our house became available. We rented this home with an option to buy at the end of a year. It was in the Oak Forest subdivision, with wide streets wonderful for walking or bike riding. Elizabeth was a third grader at Estes Elementary School down the street and Andrew was enrolled at the Sunshine Preschool just a mile from our home. We had a beautiful backyard for the kids to play, and the home had a large living room, a small kitchen, a small dining room, three bedrooms, and two baths. Once we moved into the house, it didn't seem to have enough room for active children. So after a year of renting, we moved to Hendersonville, where Keith worked at Pardee Hospital.

We started discussing having an addition to our family. However, we had a major conflict when Keith changed his mind and decided he didn't want another child. After some time, the arguments lessened but I carried anger and resentment from his change of mind.

We bought a home in Hendersonville, the first we owned since moving to Jacksonville. It was a two-story house, built in 1926, with four bedrooms, a formal living room, a dining room, a kitchen, and a sunroom. There wasn't much of a yard, but there was a city park close by where the children could play. We moved into the new home in May 1990.

Elizabeth entered fifth grade at Hendersonville Elementary school and Andrew began first grade at Bruce Drysdale. Both were happy and settled well into life in Hendersonville. I continued driving to North Buncombe while Keith continued to work at the hospital. We attended the First United Methodist Church. It seemed like things were settling down and life was going well.

CHAPTER 6

THE PREGNANCY

Dare:

In late May of 1992 I was out of school for Memorial Day. Keith and I were taking a walk by the high school when I mentioned to him that I was three days late with my period. He said, "Oh, I bet you're pregnant." I said, "No, I'm 38 years old and probably in early perimenopause." He responded, "Oh no, we're going to the drugstore to get a pregnancy test now!"

At the pharmacy, Keith inquired on the reliability of the test, and was told it was 99.9% accurate. I was so embarrassed, thinking the whole store knew what was going on and that he assumed I was positive, making a big deal out of the situation.

We returned home and I took the test. I couldn't believe it when the results were positive. I was shocked, angry, scared, and said a few choice words! I was so mad at Keith and told him, "If you had just let me have this baby earlier, I wouldn't be an old lady, would have had my tubes tied, and the baby would be in kindergarten by now!"

I'd wanted another baby several years ago, after the birth of Andrew. At first, Keith had agreed to a third child. However, he changed his mind when the time came, telling me he wanted to wait until Andrew was in kindergarten so we wouldn't have two children in daycare at the same time. But when that time came, Keith no longer wanted another child; he had changed his mind. I was so angry and felt betrayed because he had originally agreed to it. I, in turn, agreed to having my tubes tied afterward. My main goal in life was to be a mother and a teacher, but Keith thought he was too old.

This was a major stand-off between us, "How could he renege on this after I agreed to have my tubes tied?" At that time, I had told him that I would never forgive him. Now, several years later and being older, we found ourselves in this position.

After calming down, we went to Andrew's baseball game in south Asheville, acting as if nothing was happening. It was exceedingly difficult to focus on the game. When I returned to school after the holiday, I let my principal know and was incredibly stressed out. She tried to comfort me, reciting a bible verse about how God knew the baby in the womb and that everything would be fine. I said, "I don't need this baby. It's just a bad time in my life to start over when I'm a full-time teacher, wife, and mother who's also just opened a part-time costume business." It felt like more than I could handle.

The first three months of the pregnancy were stressful. Keith and I had a lot of heavy-duty conversations: "Do you want an abortion?" "What if it has Down's Syndrome?" "What about adoption?" We decided neither of us could handle abortion or adoption. We agreed we would keep the child no matter what condition it might have.

I was considered a "geriatric mother" and amniocentesis was indicated. Nobody asked if I wanted amniocentesis, but it was routinely performed on pregnant women 35 and older. The length of the needle alone was enough to make anyone pass out, and the procedure itself could result in loss of the baby. I decided not to get attached until the baby and I survived it.

We had an ultrasound done when the fetus was 11 weeks and three days old. We received a VHS tape of the baby, and could see its little nose and watch it put a hand up to its mouth to start sucking. I told Keith, "Nobody can ever tell me that this isn't a real little person." I knew I could never have an abortion, nor think of one in the same way again.

The young technician asked if we wanted to know the baby's sex. We said, "Yes," and she replied, "It looks like a boy." So for eleven days, I called the baby Jefferson and Andrew called the baby Ryan (after his little best friend). Then, while I was on the phone with Keith one day, the fluid examiner from NC-Chapel Hill beeped in to give us the results of the amniocentesis. He reported there were no signs of trouble and said it looked as if everything was fine. He asked if I wanted to know the sex and I replied, "It's a boy, right?" "No," he answered, "it's a girl." I was so excited and called Keith back right away. We were both delighted to learn that she was normal, then we calmed down and named the baby Anna Kathryn ReHazel. The name ReHazel came from the first letters of my sister, Rebecca, and my mother's name, Hazel.

In the coming nights, we talked and sang to her. She would respond to our voices, kicking and moving around. All of us became ready to welcome a new family member. We had goals for Anna: Keith wanted her to be a prissy, frilly girl, quite social. Elizabeth wanted to show her the "real world." Andrew said he was going to teach the baby her first word, and it was going to be "baseball."

My goal was to relax and enjoy this baby, since Elizabeth had been in the hospital for croup and bronchitis as an infant for several nights, and Andrew had been in for spinal meningitis for two long weeks at the age of seven months. Surely, Anna would be fine, with no major complications!

I wanted to work until I went into labor. She was due January 26, 1993. The director of personnel wanted me to start leave on January 15th, which was the beginning of the second semester when students would be better able to adjust to a substitute. I agreed to this plan.

On January 20th, I had an appointment with a doctor who was a Woody Allen look-alike. I asked to be induced early. I was tired and had been having Braxton-Hicks contractions since December. I knew the baby was full term. However, he wanted to let nature take its course and have me wait till the due date.

The next night, after the appointment, I received sad news that a fellow teacher's son had lost his battle to leukemia. This grieved me so much. On Sunday morning after church, Keith, the kids, and I were riding down Finley Cove Road from his parents' home. It was foggy and cold. Keith said I shouldn't go to the child's funeral. I replied, "I cannot imagine the agony of losing a child." As soon as I said it, Anna kicked with such force I couldn't believe its strength. When we got home, we watched TV and ate chips and salsa in our sunroom. We went to bed late and, surprisingly, didn't talk to Anna, but instead fell asleep. It was January 24.

Keith:

The morning of the 25th, Dare awoke around four a.m. to announce she was having significant pain and felt that she was in labor. She prepared herself for the trip to the hospital. I told Elizabeth and Andrew the news that their sister was on the way, and they needed to prepare for school while Dare and I went to the hospital. I called my father, Bob, to report and to make sure he was coming to take the children to school. Andrew was in third grade and Elizabeth in seventh. Bob assured me that he was on his way and would be available to assist if needed during the day.

Soon we all were ready for this special day. As Dare and I left the house, we were excited. Before leaving for the hospital, I passed the nursery, which had been prepared weeks ahead, to pick up her outfit and blanket. The nursery even had Christmas presents awaiting her arrival. As we left, I reassured the kids that I would be home to take them to the hospital as soon as their sister was born.

I had accepted the anticipation of a new family member and was extremely excited, looking forward to Anna's birth. I helped Dare to the car for the 25-minute drive to the hospital.

Dare:

All the way to Mission Hospital, I told Keith, "This doesn't feel the same as the other pregnancies," knowing that every pregnancy was different. We weren't concerned, just so excited.

Elizabeth wrote a sweet note for Keith and put it in his jacket for when the baby came. He told me it said, "Ok Mom, push! Soon you will have a beautiful baby girl. Push, Mom, push!"

When we arrived at Mission, I was taken to a room where the baby would be born. A nurse came in with a stethoscope and placed it on my stomach, moving it around several times. She looked concerned and went to get the charge nurse, Mrs. Jan, the R.N. I looked at Keith, saying, "This isn't good. They can't find the heartbeat." Jan the R.N. checked for the heartbeat, then went to get a doctor. When he came into the room, he, too, checked for a heartbeat. He looked up and spoke matter-of-factly, "I'm sorry to say you have a fetal demise."

My regular doctor showed up around seven a.m. He learned of the situation and wanted me to have an epidural. I was going to have to deliver Anna and knew it was going to be a long day. I was in shock but knew when the contractions were coming before the monitor even indicated. It was suggested I take more medication so I wouldn't have pain. I told them I could handle the pain, but they insisted.

I told Keith that I didn't want him to call my parents about the stillbirth until Anna was delivered. I did not want them worrying about me. He said that he had already called his father to inform him, but he would wait until after the delivery before calling my parents. I was very worried about our children and didn't want them to find out from their grandfather. Dr. Hicks said he could stop the delivery until the children could come to the hospital. He offered to meet with them to answer questions or help in support.

Keith left the hospital to tell the children. He first stopped to tell Elizabeth of the news. She was upset, crying, and worrying about me. Keith then went with her to tell Andrew. When they arrived at his school, he was jumping up and down, saying, "Did my sister come? Is my sister here?" Keith took him to the library and told him. He was quiet and upset.

Keith then drove them to the hospital. They came to the room to make sure I was okay. Grandma Kay-Kay was there with Grandad Bob. She took the children to the Health Adventure while I was still in the process of delivering Anna. Grandad Bob stayed in the lobby until they returned.

Dr. Hicks explained to me that Anna's neck was flexed back, with the cord wrapped around her neck twice. He made a call to the Mountain Area Health and Education Center to consult with another physician regarding the best way to deliver Anna. He didn't want to do a C-section or major surgery if he could prevent further recovery issues. It was recommended that he use a vacuum extractor. Anna was delivered weighing seven pounds and six ounces. Dr. Hicks expressed sorrow that she had bruises and some torn skin above her eye.

Jan, the R.N., was with me. She told me she had two older children and a boy, Phillip, who lived only a brief time. She knew the emotional pain I was having and wanted to be available to me. She stayed an extra four hours beyond her shift, and asked if I wanted to get up to hold and wash my baby. I said, "No," because I had never touched a dead body and wasn't sure I wanted to. I was still in shock from the whole day. Jan the R.N. took Anna out of the isolette and laid her down with care. I thought, "How can I deny her after nine months carrying her?" I told the R.N. I would hold her, and she put Anna into my arms. She told me I could keep her for as long as I wanted before they took her to the morgue.

Elizabeth and Andrew came into the room and stood by Anna. I held her for a long, long time. Then Elizabeth held her, but Andrew declined. It was about seven p.m. when I told Keith, "Let's send both the children home and Anna to the morgue." Then Andrew decided to hold her, saying, "But I didn't get to hold my little sister!" So he did.

Jan the R.N. came in, saying she would be down to see me in the morning before starting her shift. She asked if I wanted to stay on the maternity floor or go to another floor, saying some women prefer to go to another area of the hospital. However, I felt that I could handle staying on the maternity ward. Later that evening, the staff rolled me through the ward to a room at the end of the hall. I rolled past the nursery and knew I might hear babies crying, but I felt like I could handle it even though everything still seemed surreal. I didn't sleep well that night and had a CNA named Hazel, which was my mother's name, and felt some comfort.

Keith had talked earlier with my mother regarding what had happened. She was relieved I was doing okay and sorry regarding the loss. I was later able to talk with her and feel her comfort and support.

All night I kept the light on at my bed while I listened to the trains going by in the distance. I heard carts going down the hall. I was struck by the thought that everything went on around me while I felt like an isolated stranger, looking at the world from the other side. My world ended that day, but the rest of the world went on without me.

The next morning, true to her word, Jan the R.N. came to my room. She said, "Would you like a lock of Anna's hair?" and asked if I wanted to get her out of the morgue and hold her again. She warned me that Anna would be cold. I declined to hold her but wanted the lock of her dark hair. She said the chaplain, Mark, would retrieve the lock.

Jan was an earth angel. I had never met her before, but she meant so much to me. I will never forget how one person made such a difference. She even sent a dozen, baby-bud pink roses to me at home on the first-year anniversary of my loss.

Before I left the hospital, the Woody Allen look-alike doctor came by, sat down, and said he was sorry this had happened. I replied, as sadly as I possibly could, "If only you had induced me as I requested."

Keith told me later that day that he was so proud of me and how I conducted myself through the delivery, loss and all. I asked, "Why?" He said most would have screamed, cried, and yelled. I answered, "It wouldn't have brought my baby back."

Dr. Hicks told us there was no physical reason I couldn't have another baby, but he would prefer I wait a year before the next. I didn't think I would want another baby at the age of forty, with delivery at forty-one. Keith didn't object, saying we could plan for this event. The next day at home, each child snuggled next to me in bed and asked when we could have another baby.

Keith:

The shock of Anna's death was devastating. I felt numb in the delivery room when the doctor told us of her demise, my heart pounding as I looked at Dare. My mind raced with so many questions. I worried about Dare going through delivery, and her physical, emotional, and mental status. How do I tell our children? What do I say to our parents? Do we have a funeral? I wondered how this could happen when the pregnancy seemed to go so well.

I couldn't help but feel guilt thinking of all the times we argued about having another child. Was this punishment from God for all the negative things I said about having another child? Why did this occur when I had finally accepted the addition of a new baby?

As the morning progressed, I knew I had to deal with these questions. I first called my father to tell him she hadn't made it. He was emotional when he paused to tell my mother. She came on the phone, crying and asking about Dare. I told her that she was naturally upset but preparing for a long day waiting for the delivery. My mom said they would come to the hospital to help with anything they could do. I asked them to stay with our children while we waited for Anna to be delivered.

When I went back to the room with Dare, she was concerned for Elizabeth and Andrew. She talked with Dr. Hicks, who said he could hold off delivery until I could tell them and bring them to the hospital. On the way to tell the kids, I rehearsed how to approach them with the news. I continued to worry about Dare. After the initial conversation with both children and assuring them their mother was fine, we went back to the hospital so they could see for themselves. Then my parents came to stay with Elizabeth and Andrew while we waited for the delivery.

It was a long afternoon, but soon Anna came. The doctor explained it was an umbilical cord accident and there was nothing we did, or could have done, to prevent this occurrence.

Dare:

I was discharged on Tuesday. It was so strange, leaving the hospital without my baby in my arms. I couldn't believe the sadness in my heart.

Keith and his dad had already picked out a plot in the family lot for burial. They chose a tiny, white coffin with a spray of pink roses for Anna's body. We met with our minister at the First Methodist Church, where we discussed plans for burial. We had a private family viewing. Anna was so beautiful, dressed in a pink dress with a bonnet.

Elizabeth placed a gold necklace, with a half of a bible verse, on her neck. She kept the other piece around her neck. Andrew placed a stuffed little dog next to her. I had a family picture put in the coffin with writing on the back that said, "You are a special child of God. You will always be a part of our family. You will remain in our hearts and minds forever."

We scheduled the graveside service on a Friday. That morning there was snow on the ground and cold in the air. I didn't expect a lot of people to come to the service in winter, but over one hundred people showed up.

One of my co-workers, the physical education coach, was about to have his third baby. He told me that if they had twins, he would give one to us. When we received baby items in the mail afterwards, I would take them to him.

I looked up to see the face of a friend who had buried an infant son several years earlier. It was a shock, but it meant so much to feel their love and support. I will always be thankful for their kind words of sympathy.

Keith:

On Friday morning, many of our fellow peers, friends, and relatives gathered for support and the sharing of love. I remember noticing a friend, David, who lost his son to spinal meningitis at seven months, shortly after our Andrew had recovered. We had developed a friendship with this couple when our pediatrician told us about them, thinking we could offer them some support. They were in the hospital's PICU with their own Andrew, having the same illness. I went to meet them, but shortly after my visit their infant child died. Now, eight years later, David had read about Anna's death and came to the graveside service to be with us. My eyes were full of tears as we hugged.

One teacher, who taught Andrew in the first grade, was especially talented in art. She etched the picture of an angel on Anna's tombstone.

Many of friends and coworkers from my job at the hospital came to offer support and love. It was a sad, but very blessed, day as we said good-bye. Over the next several months, I remained aware of Dare's and our children's emotions, but denied my own mental health. Six months later, I was in church during the baptism of an infant and suddenly found myself engulfed in tears as I watched the baby being baptized in her father's arms at the altar.

The following months were difficult in adjustment and grief. Andrew would notice his mother crying, and often ask her, "Mom, what are you doing?" I think it was his way of letting her know we needed her. Many times, Dare said it was only due to her living children that she was able to get out of bed, knowing they needed her, and that she needed to be strong for them. However, I know she spent much thought and grief during her moments of aloneness. I remember asking her, in the darkness of the night, "Dare, where are you? Come back – you are so far away from me!" She would respond that she was sad and felt far away.

CHAPTER 7

RETURN TO SCHOOL

Dare:

I remained at home the entire six weeks of my maternity leave, choosing to do it in an effort to cope with my physical and mental self. When I returned to school, people said, "If this had to happen to anyone, it was best that it was you; you are such a strong person." While this was meant to be a compliment, I thought if this were the case, I didn't want to be strong. One fellow teacher came to ask me if I wanted to sell my baby stuff, which felt hurtful and tacky so soon after Anna's death.

The thing that encouraged me the most were the words of another teacher, who told me that she'd had a little boy who only lived a short time. He was born without kidneys, and had been her only child.

She felt she would never smile or be happy again. But then, one afternoon while driving home, she looked at the mountains and saw the sun setting. She smiled and felt a little bit of joy for the first time since her loss. She shared, "I know you may think you will never be happy again or have anything to smile about, but one day, when you least expect it, it will happen for you."

I clung to this hope. I felt she spoke the truth to me. The fact that she went through what she'd experienced gave her words credibility. She was another Earth Angel who came my way.

I completed the school year, and at that point the Hendersonville city and county school systems merged. I requested a transfer to the elementary school where our son, Andrew, was entering into a year-round program. I wanted to be on the same schedule, so I negotiated with the director of special education to teach the learning disabled and educable/mentally challenged students (but not the behavioral/emotional students). We agreed upon it, and I started the year-round program in June of 1993.

After the second day on the job, I asked the principal, "Where is the BEH teacher?" He responded, "You're it!" He'd sent the other teacher back to the administrative office feeling he didn't need two staff in special education. Then he assigned me to be the BEH teacher.

I was upset with this assignment, feeling I hadn't agreed to it. But the principal made it clear that he had the authority to make the decision, not the county office. I got caught in the crossfire, and this became another adjustment I had to make. During the next two years, I began experiencing some neurological symptoms, including the dragging of my leg, balance issues, and extreme fatigue. I wasn't sure what caused this, but noticed it seemed to happen more when I was under stress.

CHAPTER 8

BLIND? YOU'VE GOT TO BE KIDDING!

Dare:

It had really been a tumultuous year, with one thing after another. It made me eager for 1994. I told this to Keith while he was driving on the last day of the year, and he hit a pothole and blew out a tire. This year couldn't end soon enough!

In November, my friend and I planned a trip to Charlotte for the Southern Living Christmas show. On the morning we were to leave, I woke up blind in one eye. When I opened my eyes, my left eye could see nothing but pure whiteness, as if someone had put a piece of typing paper over that eye. If it had been all-black, I would've freaked out because I thought blindness would be pure darkness. But because the light in my eye was pure white, I didn't panic. I thought something else had to be causing it. I thought it would clear up, so I planned to continue with the trip to Charlotte. I cleaned my contact lenses, hoping that my vision would clear.

The phone rang and my friend said she had to cancel our trip because her child was sick. I was disappointed but thought, "That's how things happen when you have children." I thought I would just spend my day with Keith and the children. I knew I would have a good day with my family so long as there was sight in one eye; I could still enjoy activities regardless of the blindness.

By Saturday night, my vision did not clear. Keith asked if I wanted to go to the hospital to check it out. I said, "No, I'll just wait and see if it clears by morning." By the next night, I still had no sight in my left eye and began to worry, although I was still more puzzled than scared. I called my friend, Tami, who worked with me at school and whose husband worked for a prominent ophthalmologist in town. I thought her husband might give me a clue as to my loss of vision. Rob told Tami, "Oh, that's not good. Tell her to come to the office in the morning and we'll run some tests."

On Monday, Tami drove me to her husband's office. Rob hooked me up to an IV, running dye through it so he could perform scans of my eye. At each click of the camera, I felt a wave of nausea rush over me. It was horrible and made me want to throw up. Rob told me later that I did better than some people and acknowledged that many had a similar experience, even wetting themselves or throwing up. This was a test I hoped never to repeat.

After the episode with Rob, I entered the ophthalmologist's exam room where the eye charts hung on the wall. When I closed my right eye, I couldn't see a single thing on the wall, not one mark, absolutely nothing. Dr. Lowe told me he'd never seen anyone with vision this severe. He further stated that my color vision had been affected and might never return. The official diagnosis was optic neuritis. This is a condition that damages the cover of the optic nerve, which is the vital nerve fiber transmitting visual information from the eye to the brain.

The eye specialist wanted me to return in two weeks. The day before the appointment, I regained my vision after being blind in that left eye for 13 days.

But things were still off: I could look at a jacket out of my right eye and see that the color was blue. But out of the left eye, it was black. I could see out of both eyes but had a lot of double vision. This lasted for six more weeks. During this time, I continued to work and drive the short distance to Bruce Drysdale Elementary School and back home.

Most of my color vision returned, but with somewhat different pink and orange shades. Dr. Lowe told me that if I wanted a second opinion, I might want to consult a neurologist. I followed up by scheduling an appointment with a neurologist for December 28, 1994. Keith would attend the appointment with me.

I dreaded the upcoming Christmas holidays without Anna. I wanted to get out of town and didn't feel comfortable with the usual trip to my parents' home. My brother and his wife had just delivered their baby girl in August, and I couldn't bear seeing her. This would be the first time in my life I didn't visit them during the holidays. I got on the phone with a travel agency to see what they had to offer. The agent said, "It would be cheaper to take your family on a cruise rather than Walt Disney World. For the same cost, you could fly out of Asheville to Fort Lauderdale and take a cruise to the Bahamas." I scheduled the trip for December 17th through the 21st, hoping to possibly become pregnant on the cruise.

I fully believe it was a God-thing when, on December 9, there was a cancellation at the neurologist's office. The receptionist called me at school and said, "Dr. Menn has a cancelled appointment this afternoon. Would you like to take it?" I said, "Oh, yes, I'd be happy to come in today." I then called Keith, who was at work, to ask if he could join me. Unfortunately, he couldn't attend.

I asked some of my friends around school if they knew anything about optic neuritis. The physical therapist finally said, "I'm not sure, but I think it has something to do with lupus or multiple sclerosis." I cringed inside. The idea of having a crippling muscle disease seemed like one of the worst things I could imagine. I was definitely going to ask the neurologist about this!

That afternoon I saw Dr. Menn, the neurologist, and asked about optic neuritis as it related to what my friend said. Did it have anything to do with MS or lupus? The doctor looked at me and said, "Well, we don't usually tell our optic neuritis patients this, but since you asked, I might as well lay the cards on the table. About 50% of optic neuritis patients do return with a diagnosis of multiple sclerosis." I began to cry and he snapped at me, "Well, it's not terminal!"

I left his office very shaken up. I thought, "There goes our baby. I don't want to bring a child into the world if I can't be a proper mother and take care of it." This was a close call; if I hadn't had the appointment on that earlier date, there was a good chance I would have become pregnant on the cruise.

Later that afternoon, I met Keith at the middle school where Elizabeth was having a dance. As soon as he saw me he came to the car and asked, "What did the doctor say?" I broke into tears again, saying, "We can't have another baby." He said, "Did the doctor say that?" I said, "Half of the patients with this come back with multiple sclerosis. I want to take care of the baby; I don't want the baby to take care of me."

Then I stated, "Please don't tell anybody what I just told you. It'll be grounds for divorce if you tell anyone about this conversation." I especially didn't want our children concerned or worried that their mother might end up crippled. I just felt we would let things turn out the way they would. I didn't want to address the baby situation, nor why I didn't want to have another child.

Keith:

Upon learning of Dare's blindness, I was overly concerned. I didn't push her to go to the hospital because she wanted to see if the eye would clear up on its own. However, when it continued, I was relieved she followed up with the eye specialist. I also supported her decision to make an appointment with the neurologist to gain a second opinion on the issue.

When she reported this might have something to do with multiple sclerosis, I was very worried. I didn't know much about this disease, nor how this diagnosis might change things for our family. I was especially concerned for Dare, having seen her go through the stress of Anna's death and her desire for another child. When she told me this dream was shattered, I felt so much grief. I understood she'd always wanted to be a mother, and this would have been her last attempt.

I was surprised when she told me she didn't want to have another child. Knowing how much we had disagreed before Anna, this was a remarkable choice, but I understood why she didn't want to be in a position where she couldn't offer that child her full attention, nor care for it the way she wanted, if she were to have MS.

We had gone through _____ over the past year and things were just beginning to feel more stable. Because of my profession as a social worker, I thought I could handle anything that would come our way if MS became our reality.

CHAPTER 9

SYMPTOMS PERSIST

Dare:

After Christmas, I returned to Bruce Drysdale. I remember one day when my speech became slurred. It went away after a few minutes, so I ignored it. But I didn't think it was good. In addition to the episode with my speech, I had some problems with weakness in my leg. These physical difficulties were concerning, but I didn't allow them to disrupt my desire to teach.

I loved most of my students. Some were extremely sweet and worked hard. I did not like having to be so firm, consistent, and tough with one BEH student, who was in second grade. He was the child who spit in my eye at one point, in addition to not following my directions. He distracted other students, who also had behavioral problems, with disruptions in the classroom. When I referred this one student to the office, the principal and his teacher felt he was too disruptive in the regular classroom and needed to come to me for half days. I started thinking I would have this student for the next three years, and I couldn't take it any longer; it was affecting my health.

One afternoon, I told my principal I needed to go to the county office to meet with the director of special education. When I arrived asking for a conference, her receptionist said, "No, she's busy in a meeting." I told her, "Well, I'll wait for her." I sat in the waiting room until she was available, then told her that I needed out of the BEH assignment. I reminded her that I never agreed to the position, and my stress and health were of concern. I said if she didn't find me another job, I would be out on disability and the school system would pay for it. Not only that, but they would have to pay for someone to replace me. She agreed to do what she could.

A few days later, I received a telephone call from the director of personnel. He informed me that there was a Chapter One reading position for which I could interview at my old school at Hillandale. I agreed to an interview. However, when I went to meet with the principal of the school, he said the job had been changed from a Chapter One position to a first grade classroom. I said I wasn't sure I was certified to teach first grade. However, I then recalled I had obtained the certification when I was teaching in South Carolina. We both agreed this would be a good match for me and I was offered the position.

Before starting my new job, I still had one day at Bruce Drysdale. During lunch in the cafeteria with Andrew's fourth grade teacher, she told me Andrew was so bright he needed more of a challenge, one she couldn't give him because she was busy teaching to the norm of the class and couldn't come up with extra things to meet his needs. She said if he were her child, she would consider a transfer for him to Immaculata Catholic school. I said to her, "Are you kidding me? You, being the daughter of the superintendent, would move him to a private school?" She said, "Yes, I would."

After that conversation, I went home and talked with Keith. We decided to enroll Andrew in the nearby Catholic school. This meant Andrew would have the summer off from the year-round program and start the year at Immaculata in the fall of '94. Andrew started his new class with 16 students. He loved his teacher and made some great friends. About three weeks into the year, he asked if he could walk to meet Elizabeth after school, then come together to my school. He wanted to start walking with his friend, Beau, who walked every day to the high school to meet his mother, who was also a teacher. I said that would be fine.

On the first day I allowed him to walk, both kids were late arriving. I heard an ambulance in the distance, which seemed to come toward my school's direction. I panicked, hearing the sirens and police cars, thinking something had happened. I left school and tried to walk in the direction they would be coming. I heard other students passing me, saying a boy was hit by a car while walking across the highway. My heart began to pound; I was so afraid Andrew had been struck.

I noticed my leg weakening and couldn't walk without extreme difficulty due to being anxious. The more I tried to run, the harder it became. Suddenly a car passed with a young man I knew. He yelled out his window, "Ms. Ford, it's not Andrew who was hit!" Apparently, the friend who was walking with Andrew stepped out into the street and was hit.

This child was the one taken to the hospital. When I found Andrew sitting on the sidewalk, I tried to run to hold him tight, but my legs couldn't respond quickly. Andrew appeared concerned for his friend, but remained quiet. I was just so grateful that he was all right, but I realized something was seriously happening to my health.

Keith:

Dare came home and told me of the day's events with Andrew walking to the school, and I was relieved to hear he was okay. I was concerned about Beau and talked with his parents, and learned he escaped major injury. His mom expressed concern for both boys, and we were relieved to learn they were okay, just frightened.

I was more concerned to hear about Dare's leg. I'd been worried off and on when she had similar episodes of leg weakness and fatigue while walking. I asked if she felt the need to seek medical attention to determine what was going on with her health. For some time, I'd thought she had damage from the birth of Anna, and perhaps some of these episodes were a result of the pregnancy. She didn't feel that her condition had anything to do with Anna.

I asked her again about her seeing a doctor, and she stated, "When I am strong enou   e a bad diagnosis, then I will see a doctor. I'm so   ef from the loss of Anna, the possibility of havin_   r the optic neuritis, the realization of not having another baby, and the stress of my job. I'm not ready to get a negative report. Don't ask the question if you can't take the answer."

I realized I couldn't force her and had to accept that she was simply not ready.

CHAPTER 10

TIME FOR THE ANSWER

Keith:

Dare started her new job back at Hillandale as a first-grade teacher. I helped her set up the classroom and organize her teaching materials. Her school year went well with the students and parents. She seemed to love her position and had less stress after working with the BEH population.

I was still concerned about her overall health in that she continued having weakness in her left leg. She seemed in denial about the symptoms and wanted to put her energy into establishing her classroom. When I asked how she was feeling, she always said, "Just fine," and ignored my concern. I really felt something was going on but knew I wasn't able to do anything to convince her to seek medical attention until she was ready to accept the outcome. For most of the '94-95 school year, she continued focusing on her class.

One morning in the fall of 1995 she fell while going to her car, the first major fall from losing her balance. I helped pick her up from the ground. She finally said, "I'm ready to see a doctor and find out what's going on with me."

Within the week, she made an appointment with a family physician I knew from the hospital. Dr. Ball suggested an MRI to assist getting in a clear diagnosis and scheduled an appointment for later that month at the Asheville MRI center. Due to her fear of the procedure he prescribed valium, which she began taking while we sat in the waiting room. After the third pill, and her stress level still being high, I finally took the bottle away from her for fear she would overdose!

I escorted her to the exam room where, at her insistence, she asked me to sit at the end of the table while the tests were completed. We were both nervous, but I was glad that she had finally agreed to pursue an answer to her situation.

The MRI was completed and reports sent to Dr. Ball. I received a telephone call at my work. I wasn't sure why he called me rather than Dare, but I was scared, my heart beating fast and anxiety increasing. He began the conversation by saying, "I am sorry to report that the test results indicate a diagnosis of MS." Dare had 12 lesions on the brain, which were an indicator of the disease. He continued by saying he had just met Dare and didn't know her well enough to determine the best way to share this information. I said that I would let her know. He wanted to talk with both of us that afternoon.

I wasn't totally surprised by the findings, but concerned about how this would change our family. I did not know the course of the illness nor how either of us would respond. I knew it would be a change to the overall relationship. For 20 years we had been busy with our goals of education, careers, moves, and rearing children. We had an exceptionally good marriage overall. Since 1993 – with the death of Anna, optic neuritis, stress on the job, the change in her health, and now this diagnosis of MS – everything seemed to be changing in our lives. I was scared, fearing the unknown and how this would impact our lives.

I drove slowly to her school, while fearing how I was going to tell her. I stopped at the office, my hands shaking and heart pounding. I told the receptionist of the news and my need to speak with Dare. She told me that while

Dare was in a faculty meeting, I could interrupt due to the circumstances.

Dare:

When we went to the MRI on Tuesday night they told me I would have the results back by Friday. So when I looked up and saw Keith motioning me out of the faculty meeting on Wednesday afternoon, I was incredibly surprised. I protested, somewhat nervously, being called out of a faculty meeting, "What are you doing here? You're going to get me in trouble." He said, "I just came to see my wife. Can't I see my wife?"

He walked me down the hallway into my classroom. It never crossed my mind he might have the MRI results. It had been less than 24 hours, so I wasn't anticipating any results. When we went to the classroom, he wanted me to sit down across from him, then told me Dr. Ball had called. He said that the results from the MRI confirmed a diagnosis of MS. He then started to cry. I said, "Why are you crying?"

Keith tearfully said, "Because I love you and I don't want you to have this." I replied, "Well, it could be worse. It could have been a brain tumor." I really did think it could have been a brain tumor and was relieved when it wasn't. I did know that something was wrong because of my off-and-on symptoms over the past 23 months: the tingling in the arms, electrical shocks in my leg, weakness in my legs when stressed, when I fell from balance issues, the time my throat closed, and another when my speech slurred.

Now, with this confirmed diagnosis, I wondered about the multitude of other incidents I had ignored. I recalled a time several years ago when a big German Shepherd ran out in front of my car as I was on my way to school in Asheville. When I stopped to deal with the situation, my legs were jumping up and down as I sat in the car. I had to wait till they settled down before I could proceed to work.

Another time, on a workday, I didn't hear the principal calling me on the intercom. When a couple of teachers told me he had called several times, I became incredibly stressed and my left arm began tingling vigorously. I had to physically hold it to get the arm to stop. A teacher who saw this said I needed to go to a neurologist, but I didn't take her seriously because I got over it.

One other time, when Keith and I were walking to a staff Christmas party at the hospital, I was carrying a large glass bowl with party mix and fell, cutting my hand and skinning my knee. At the time of this accident, I didn't think anything about it.

Thinking back on these incidents, I now believe I was having early symptoms of MS.

We left immediately for Dr. Ball's office, and he explained the situation to us. He said, "I am so sorry about this. There is no cure for it now, but I know they're doing research. I do want you to see a neurologist." I said, "Well, I don't want to go back to Dr. Menn." He replied, "I can refer you to Dr. Perkins in Asheville instead." I told him, "If there is no cure or medication for it, just send me a postcard when they have one." I'm not sure he liked my sense of humor.

I saw Dr. Perkins at the end of December 1995. Using his words, he felt MS was "just a nuisance," with symptoms coming and going (indicating a relapsing/remitting diagnosis). I thought I could handle it. Afterall, I was as strong as anyone else; I could deal with this.

Keith:

There were no medications approved for treatment at the time of Dare's diagnosis. Sadly, during the coming months of January and February of '96, she continued to have problems with fatigue and walking and dragging her left leg. Soon she had to use a cane. Our afternoon walks around the neighborhood were interrupted by the need to stop and rest before proceeding.

I became concerned with our health insurance coverage. I was under Dare's policy but not sure of future coverage, so I made the decision to apply for a state position to ensure health insurance. I accepted a job as a family therapist with Trend Mental Health Center, seeing adolescents and working with their parents. I was assigned to the satellite clinic in Brevard and traveled the 18 miles from Hendersonville to Brevard each day.

After several months, with no change in her physical condition, it was recommended that Dare seek a specialist in the area of MS. We attempted to contact Dr. Kemp, who was the director of the MS center in Charlotte. An appointment wasn't available for four months, so we scheduled it for July of '96. Meanwhile, it became more obvious the symptoms were increasing. On one occasion, Dare stumbled and dropped a plate of spaghetti on the floor while carrying the meat sauce to the table.

I took on more of the household duties such as cleaning, shopping, laundry, and childcare responsibilities. At the same time, we both downplayed the symptoms as much as we could to protect the kids from worry. As Dare's health declined, I felt I needed to be closer to home and more available to our children. I accepted a position in our community hospital as a medical social worker. I was assigned to all areas of the hospital, including the emergency room, ICU, labor/delivery, and medical surgery. My cases involved more complex patients with medical needs at discharge: substance abuse, child neglect/abuse, domestic concerns, adoptions, discharge planning, and locating families of unclaimed bodies at death.

The new position gave me a wealth of experience in helping resolve medical and psychological issues, but at home I felt unable to resolve the health concerns of my wife. This was a difficult reality to accept. I knew I could give the love and support necessary for her medical needs, but feared the unknown aspects of her underlying condition.

July finally came, and we traveled to Charlotte to see Dr. Kemp in hopes of finding answers.

CHAPTER 11

CHARLOTTE CENTER

Keith:

Upon arrival at the Charlotte MS center, we were anxious and scared of the potential findings. But knew we needed more substantial answers than those which the first neurologist gave us when he thought the symptoms would subside. We met Dr. Kemp who upon completing his evaluation, said, "Dare, I don't think you're taking this diagnosis seriously. I'm concerned you're progressing quickly and if you don't do something soon, you may end up in a vegetative state."

We were both surprised by his comments. Dare responded, "Well, Dr. Perkins said MS was just a nuisance, so I felt I could live with the diagnosis. The other neurologist told me it wasn't terminal...so I believed him when he said this was just an inconvenience." These conflicting opinions had given us a false sense of hope.

Dr. Kemp felt Dare had the chronic secondary progressive form of MS, not the relapsing/remitting version, and needed to seek immediate intervention. However, with no known medication approved to stop the progression, I was confused, shocked, and disheartened. Did this mean death? How would this affect our time together, our children, our careers, and our life? We were left with an unknown future.

Dare mentioned a medication called Avonex to Dr. Kemp. It was a beta interferon supposedly approved for relapsing/remitting MS, which was coming available to the public later that fall. Because of her physical decline and his secondary progress diagnoses, he didn't recommend Avonex. However, he did recommend we see Dr. Sims, director of the MS clinic at Shepherd Center in Atlanta, saying he might diagnose her with relapsing/remitting, which would give her the opportunity to try Avonex.

Dare and I discussed the possibility of going to Atlanta. I thought if there wasn't a medication approved for secondary progressive multiple sclerosis, we had nothing to lose by going to Atlanta and hoped we could be approved for Avonex. Dr. Kemp referred us to the MS clinic in Atlanta. The first available appointment was scheduled for November, four months away.

That would be another long wait. During that time, I continued to worry about her condition. I was aware of her decline but not sure how to support her. My thoughts centered on what Dr. Kemp said about a "vegetable-like" condition. The realization that she may end up this way overwhelmed me. I felt I had to stay strong and positive for her and the kids. I wasn't even sure how to talk with her.

I initially thought the leg-dragging was related to a neurological problem which had maybe occurred during Anna's birth. I guess I was trying to find reasons to not face the truth. Some may call this living in denial, but I had to keep hoping, had to keep my mind calm.

Dare:

When first diagnosed with MS in November '95, I wasn't completely shocked. I had been suffering from some form of neurological complications for over a year and half, starting with the tingling and dragging of my leg. It was becoming more obvious that my balance was off and my energy was low.

I was more relieved upon hearing the diagnosis, having originally thought it was a brain tumor.

I had experienced earlier issues with tingling and numbness in my hands, and saw a hand specialist who diagnosed me in April of 1993 with carpal tunnel syndrome in both hands. However, I elected not to have surgery at that time; I wanted to first try wearing splints to see if they would alleviate some of the pain. Later in that fall I was diagnosed with the optic neuritis after waking one morning blind in my left eye. When it didn't clear after two days, I became more concerned.

Then I heard that optic neuritis could somehow be related to multiple sclerosis. I asked about this when meeting with the specialist and he told me how 50% of his patients were later diagnosed with MS. I was devastated and tearful about this. I wanted to become pregnant again after the loss of Anna but a diagnosis of MS would change that. I didn't want to bring a child into the world if I couldn't care for it.

While the optic neuritis did finally clear, I wasn't ready to explore the diagnosis of MS. I still experienced too much grief over the loss of the baby and didn't feel I could handle the additional news of MS. I wasn't ready to accept it.

However, I continued to have some neurological abnormalities with my walking and balance. I remained in my job teaching even while these symptoms occurred. Finally, after falling while going to my car one morning, I could no longer deny that something was majorly wrong.

We followed up with a physician who ordered an MRI and the diagnosis of MS was confirmed. While upset with this news, I was thankful – again – that it wasn't a brain tumor. I felt I could handle the MS diagnosis better.

When we went to the MS Center in Charlotte, I liked Dr. Kemp just fine, but was taken aback when he diagnosed me with secondary progressive MS. This was disappointing, but at that point I was still walking. And I guess because I'm a positive person I thought, "I'm not a vegetable yet!"

Dr. Kemp said he felt I'd shown signs of MS back when Andrew was 18 months old and I had the tingling in my arms. I still thought there was hope; I even thought he might be wrong in his diagnosis. It was hard to believe someone could look at me and suggest I was going to be a vegetable. I left Charlotte disappointed by the ▓▓▓t diagnosis, but felt hopeful at the prospe▓▓▓ng down to Atlanta to meet with the head of ▓▓▓▓▓ center there. I thought if I truly had the secondary progressive form of MS, my future would go downhill all the way; there would be no stopping the progression. I could not – and would not – believe I would become a vegetable. I would put my faith in God and Atlanta.

CHAPTER 12

ATLANTA CENTER

Keith:

When we met with Dr. Sims at the Shepherd Center in Atlanta, he began the conversation with, "It's a wonderful time to have MS!" While he might think so, I didn't feel it was such a wonderful time. I'm not sure he understood the emotional trauma we faced, given such devastating news with fear of the unknown. We were receiving conflicting messages: that her illness was "not terminal" to "it's just a nuisance" to "you're not taking this illness seriously." And now: "It's a wonderful time to have MS!" These disparate comments only led to more confusion and anxiety. I guess Dr. Sims was trying to be encouraging, hoping a cure might be coming soon.

We discussed the use of Avonex for relapsing/remitting MS with Dr. Sims. After he examined Dare, he was willing to give us a diagnosis of relapsing/remitting to pave the way for trying Avonex. We decided to follow back up with the Shepherd Center and give the new medication a chance to work.

When the Avonex became available, Dr. Sims sent the prescription to her primary physician, Dr. Ball, in Hendersonville. We scheduled the first injection on a Friday afternoon so she would have the weekend to recover in the event of side effects. The injection went deep into the muscle of the hip, and I was present so I could learn how to administer the injection at home. Dare remained at his office for a while afterward to see whether she would have a reaction. She didn't experience anything at the office, however that night she had severe side effects with the flu-like symptoms of headache, chills, fever, and weakness. These subsided within the first 24 hours.

We would often play a game when the time came for the injection. I would tease her and act as if I were chasing her around the room to give her the shot. She would try to run away, yelling, "No! No!" I would laugh and finally corner her to give the injection. The first couple of times, she wasn't able to get out of bed due to the side effects, and would take the day off from school to rest. After the initial adjustment, she was able to return to the classroom, but often with headaches.

This routine continued for several months. I tried to support her by increasing my help with household chores, providing care to her, and relieving much of the daily stressors. We also had the children involved in schoolwork and social activities needing our attention. Life was stressful trying to adjust to the changes in routine in our daily lives, but we managed.

In addition to monthly trips to Atlanta, Dare was required to undergo lab/blood tests several times a month on the third, eleventh, and 21st days after the medication to check blood levels. It got funny after that when, at the registration desk, staff members always asked the same questions: did we have insurance, did we have a weapon, what was our religion, who was our doctor, and did we have advance directives on file? After several trips, I decided to break the routine and answer these questions differently. One month I would say we were "Baptist," the next month "Jewish," and the following time we were "Methodist." I might tell them, "I left my weapon at home," or, "in the car." The lady at the desk, who was familiar with my answers, just laughed.

In addition to the monthly blood draws, Dare also received IV steroids to address any issues with inflammation and infection. This involved going to Dr. Ball's office during breaks from school to receive the IV before returning to her classroom. The infusions lasted for several months during the scheduled trips to Atlanta. With all the blood drawn from the veins, it became difficult to obtain blood without several attempts.

Dare:

As we progressed with the series of referrals, we received conflicting advice along the way: The neurologist called it a "nuisance" disease. The MS specialist who felt the opposite saying I wasn't "taking this disease seriously" and that I was declining quickly. Then the director of the MS Center at Shepherd Clinic in Atlanta, who agreed to diagnose me with relapsing/remitting MS so we could pursue the Avonex medication.

Initially, when meeting Dr. Sims in Atlanta, I was excited to be approved for the Avonex injection. The one thing that struck me was a big chart on his wall that gave the disability ratings of MS. The chart rated the disability from 1-10 at half increments. I was already at a "six" on the chart, that I could walk 25 feet unassisted. The chart indicated that "ten" was death.

At this point, I was still optimistic. I felt that the clinic in Atlanta gave me more hope. I appreciated the fact that Dr. Sims was willing to try the new medication and hoped I truly had the relapsing/remitting MS. The goal was remission.

My primary doctor didn't want me chasing after rainbows, but I was desperate. I had sought out integrative medicine and holistic approaches prior to accepting this final diagnosis. I told myself, "This illness may take my body, but it won't take my happiness." I'd already spent so much time in grief over Anna's death and losing her was worse than this illness.

Avonex came with terrible side effects that included headaches and flu-like symptoms that kept me in bed for 24 hours at a time. I wasn't pleased with these symptoms but always believe our minds are powerful and we can deal with the unpleasantness if we are hopeful.

Well, after many months of this routine, I didn't improve and became discouraged. Dr. Sims told us he didn't feel Avonex was getting the results he wanted. He then introduced the idea of adding chemotherapy to my treatment. At first, I wasn't in favor of it, but later thought of my children. I know a lady whose mother died at the age of 39 from MS. The daughter is still angry because she felt her mom gave up and didn't fight. I didn't want my children to believe that I didn't fight to stay alive for my family.

Dr. Sims said, "You don't have to decide today. If you want to go home and think about it, that's ok. Just let me know your decision." I said, "No, I'll do the chemotherapy."

Keith said, "Are you sure, Dare? Do you want to think about it?" I replied, "No, I want to go ahead and do it. Let's just set it up today." The thought of chemotherapy scared me. I wondered if I would lose all my hair and if I would be nauseated all the time. But I knew I needed to do the treatment regardless of my fears. We set the appointment up before we left the center. I was extremely quiet the whole three-and-a-half hours driving home. I kept thinking that, in addition to continuing Avonex, chemotherapy was the only other thing available to me. And while he thought the Avonex might still help, it was all a gamble. Thus far, it hadn't worked.

Dr. Sims said he thought the chemo would put me

into remission within four to nine months. I thought if I were lucky, I could accomplish that goal within his timeframe. I could certainly stand four trips to Atlanta if it meant getting me into remission. If I weren't so lucky, I felt certain I would be there within nine months. "One step at a time," I told myself.

When we went to Atlanta for my first chemo treatment, I was at the hospital from 8 a.m. to 1 p.m. We spent the night at the Piedmont Guest Room offered by the hospital for $40 dollars a night. This was so much better than the $140 dollars at the nearby motel, where we'd stayed before.

This became our routine: The night before chemotherapy, after working all day and traveling in the evening hours, we could hardly wait to get to the accommodations. We would stop at Lenox Square Mall to order Japanese food to go, eat our food, and go to bed. The next morning, we would head to the hospital. I would be hooked to an IV of saline solution, a bag of steroids, and a pouch of Cytoxan. I had to drink a gallon of water and be catheterized. Keith would stay with me and bring music to play.

After four months, I wasn't lucky enough to be in remission. This was difficult because after each trip,

I was exhausted and my energy was extremely low. I remember one time, when Keith asked me to simply sit on the front porch with him, I told him I didn't have the energy.

We made the decision to continue the chemo treatments. After the ninth session, Dr. Sims stated, "Dare, you're still not in remission. I guess we'll have to keep going."

I felt I had no choice but to continue. If I didn't go into remission, I was frightened I might become a "vegetable," like Dr. Kemp mentioned in Charlotte. Each month we continued, I didn't think I could commit to the trip and six hours of treatment. I was so drained; it wasn't easy to do this. All I could say to myself was, "For this month, I will go." I couldn't let myself think any further than one month at a time. I continued for a total of nineteen months in Atlanta. On one of those trips, I had blood in my stool and Dr. Sims withheld treatment until I went home and had a colonoscopy. I was diagnosed with ulcerative colitis, although it didn't interfere with my chemo regimen.

Finally, I asked Dr. Sims if I could continue treatment with an oncologist in Hendersonville, and he approved the request. I knew of an oncologist named Dr. Morris, who had a good reputation with her patients. Keith and I spoke with her, and she agreed to follow me in Hendersonville.

Dr. Morris remained in direct contact with Dr. Sims, and I was happy to remain home during treatment. Being in Hendersonville meant I wouldn't need to be catheterized, nor would I need to drink the gallon of water. However, Dr. Morris did make me drink two doses of some nasty-tasting liquid after each chemo. She continued to increase the dose of Cytoxan in coordination with Dr. Sims, feeling the amount given wasn't sufficient to put me in remission. She continued to increase until I reached my "lifetime limit." While I didn't go into remission after ten months, I was still alive.

One of the months, I got shingles. Dr. Morris met me at my van to give me a prescription of Acyclovir. She said, "If you aren't better in three days, I'm putting you in the hospital." I rebelled, "No, I can't go to the hospital. My parents and sister are coming this weekend to visit. I can't go." Dr. Morris replied, "I don't care. If you aren't better, I'm putting you in the hospital." Fortunately, I didn't have to be hospitalized. On the last trip I made to Atlanta, I walked in with the assistance of a walker. I looked at the disability chart on the wall and   rised to see that I had gone from a "6" to a   er a two-year period. The next step was de........ I was still determined not to move to a 10!

CHAPTER 13

DECISION TO RETIRE

Keith:

During this time, Dare continued to teach but had more problems with walking and fatigue. She started using a cane to assist with balance while in the classroom. She told me when the principal called for a fire drill, it was all she could do to escort the children from the classroom to the designated area outside. She eventually had her assistant escort the kids, while she saved her energy by hiding in the bathroom!

One day a student came to class and went to give her a big hug. Dare said, "Honey, you better be careful not to knock us to the ground." The student continued giving her a hug, causing Dare to lose balance. They both fell to the floor. Luckily neither were hurt; just embarrassed.

In spring, Dare and I visited her parents' home for Easter holiday. While there, s   ıer sister-in-law of her difficulty maintaining   n the classroom. The sister-in-law suggested .... consider applying for disability. Dare returned home and gave serious thought to this suggestion. It was hard for her to consider; her lifelong desire to be a teacher began at the age of five. But it was becoming too difficult. She had concerns about being able to safely manage her classroom structure. She decided it would be best to retire before further decline, and before the parents of her students complained about her condition. She would rather leave the classroom while still standing on her feet than face further physical decline.

She applied for Social Security Disability. While this process is usually denied on first request, it was apparent that, given the medical documentation, treatment, and continued increase in physical limitations, her case was accepted. Dare retired in the spring of 1997.

CHAPTER 14

CHILDREN

Keith:

In the midst of Dare's illness, we were actively rearing our two children, Elizabeth and Andrew. At the time of Anna's death, Elizabeth was in middle school and Andrew was in elementary. Both children were doing well in school and were involved in other activities such as dance, baseball, swimming, gymnastics, and art. They were a strong part of our family unit and seemed very normal in their childhood experiences, enjoying friends and home life.

However, I became more concerned about their reaction to Anna's death and how they would handle their mom's health. Being a social worker involved in the mental health of clients, I was especially sensitive to the emotional stability of my children. Elizabeth seemed more verbal expressing her feelings. She is more like me in that she is intuitive and expressive in her feelings and perception of things.

Andrew has always been more private sharing his thoughts. However, he's a very deep thinker and sensitive to issues. I asked his school counselor to talk with him regarding the death of Anna and the events at home. He was terribly upset with me for doing this. He told me he didn't want to talk about his "feelings" and didn't want to share thoughts about Anna or his mom.

I've wanted a close relationship with Andrew. Having been especially sensitive and expressive in my feelings, I've never felt he wanted to reciprocate. I'm not sure I have always been the father he wanted. He is more interested in sports, and I never had a father who spent time with me in those areas. However, I've tried to support Andrew in his interests and attend practices when he had baseball, football, or basketball. While I love him and wanted that expressive communication, I feel he's wanted to keep his thoughts to himself.

Over the years, I have been especially aware of our children's progress and accomplishments. I know they've been caring and concerned over their mother's health and how I've dealt with my role as caregiver, spouse, and father. Despite these concerns, they appeared to live as "normal" as possible, given the numerous appointments, treatments, and trips to Atlanta. I believe we maintained a stable environment for their development.

Elizabeth started high school during the earlier time of Dare's trips to Atlanta. Being a young, adolescent girl, it was hard to tell what effect the death of her sister and her mother's failing health had on her. She expected us to have another baby after Anna died and was furious when we chose not to pursue becoming pregnant. She later told us she felt betrayed by this. We didn't tell her the reason for changing our minds at the time, and she didn't reveal her anger until later.

While she did well in academics during those high school years, I became more concerned over her social activities. She began dating an older male who was five years her senior and had many problems. She seemed infatuated with his attention, and the relationship continued through her senior year. We were concerned she might decide not to pursue her education after high school due to his influence.

However, Elizabeth did apply to college and was accepted to her school of choice. She started at Appalachian State University in the fall of 1998 with a major in political science and plans to enter law school. She changed her mind after completing an internship at a law firm and observing the legal actions of the courtroom. She questioned the ethical decisions made. Her mother always thought she would make a good teacher, and Elizabeth pursued her teaching certificate as well as a masters in American government. She graduated with honors in both her undergraduate and graduate studies, and secured employment with the Buncombe County school system along with her national teaching certification.

In 2011, Elizabeth married Michael, who was originally employed with a CPA firm. Having always had an interest in physical rehabilitation, he decided to pursue a Ph.D. in physical therapy and now works as a physical therapist. They have three daughters.

Andrew was an avid bike rider during his middle grade years. I had an adult friend, also highly active in riding, who told me of a fundraiser for multiple sclerosis research. It was a 150-mile bike ride from the middle of North Carolina to Myrtle Beach, South Carolina. He wanted to know if Andrew might be interested in joining him, and told us he would supervise him during the ride. I spoke with Andrew, and he was excited to attempt the ride and raise money for his mother's illness. At the time he was only 12 years old.

We went along with this adventure on the condition he promise to listen to my friend and be incredibly careful. He solicited money from various friends, coaches, teachers, and church members and raised $1,200 for his team. He started the ride in Rockingham, N.C. and rode the first 70 miles to a camping space at a high school. The next morning he completed the ride to the beach. Dare and I followed his route by car, checking on his status and health. We met him at Myrtle Beach the next afternoon. We were so excited to see his bike rolling down to the finish line. He was very tired but proud of his accomplishment. He asked if we would allow him to do the ride again the following year. We agreed and he had four other boys join, with our friend supervising. He completed the second year and raised over $2,500 dollars.

In hindsight, Dare and I didn't realize how dangerous this event could be. Participants ride on back roads, highways, and places of heavy traffic. I'm not positive the organizers of this fundraiser supervised things as well as they should have. There could have been more accidents. This event has now been cancelled. We're very thankful for Andrew's contribution, and also for his safety.

We continued to encourage his participation in school studies and sports. He was an excellent student in high school and a member of the National Honor Society. He was also involved in sports, playing baseball, basketball, and soccer. All in all, an ideal teenager causing us little concern. Upon graduating from high school in 2002, he was accepted on early admission to the University of North Carolina at Chapel Hill. His major was in communications, where he was an honor student. Upon graduation, he worked with a manufacturing company and is now in an administrative position.

In 2007 Andrew announced, to our shock, that he had gotten someone pregnant. We weren't happy about this situation; the woman was several years younger and already had another child, who was two years old at the time. Our first grandson, Gavin, was born July 13, 2008. Andrew moved in with the mother but soon realized she had emotional and mental health issues and wasn't able to give the needed attention to the children. He eventually left her and, along with his son, moved in with us. He went to court to obtain joint custody and has been the predominant parent.

Andrew and Gavin lived in an Asheville apartment when he entered his master's program in business administration. He worked during the day and attended classes at night, so I often babysat Gavin while he was in school. Andrew finished his MBA in the winter of 2014, and then obtained certification as a project management specialist through an online program with Villanova University.

Several years later, Andrew began dating another lady, one who had gone to high school with him and was a year younger. When Porshe was in eighth grade, she took dance lessons, and one afternoon Andrew asked his mom if she knew her. At that young age, Andrew expressed interest and said, "She's mighty fine!" Of course, at the time, he never expected they would later meet and begin dating. In 2015, Andrew married Porshe. She has another child from a previous relationship, and they've managed to blend the boys in addition to having a child of their own.

Given the circumstances, I'm enormously proud of our children. Both Elizabeth and Andrew have completed master's programs, work in professional jobs, married good spouses, and given us seven terrific grandchildren.

I don't think either of our children have known how to help their mother. They express concern for her health and try to assist in grocery shopping, writing, and ordering items through the internet. They give moral support to their mom, but I think it is Dare that gives them inspiration, encouragement, and support. She encourages them to live their own lives without being consumed by her illness. Dare never wanted her children to stop their activities. She tried to protect them so they could live a normal adolescent life.

She continues to remain optimistic and seldom shares her inner struggles and fears that might concern others in their daily lives. For the most part, I have been the one she relies upon to share her feelings and thoughts. Although it's hard, I continue to be amazed at how she's accepted the limitations of her physical decline with such grace and courage. I am also amazed how I have continued, through the hard times and struggles, to remain in the role of her caregiver. We both have grown with this experience.

Dare:

I feel it is important for children to have a joyful and secure foundation. From the beginning, I didn't want my multiple sclerosis diagnosis to rob my children of a normal childhood. Children learn coping skills from their parents. If the parents are anchored solidly, then the children are more likely to be anchored as well. I've taught my children to let God be their best friend because He can always be there for them when others cannot. I've also acknowledged that life has its ups and downs. I have confidence they can weather the storms.

CHAPTER 15

INTERVENTIONS

Keith:

Dare actively participated in physical therapy, necessary to maintain flexibility and strength in her muscles. Her insurance paid for much of this intervention, although soon Dare was paying more because the insurance felt she wasn't progressing in her goals and classified her as "custodial care." I was upset with this decision; I felt she needed this activity to preserve her muscle strength. She eventually decided to pay $50 a month to use the equipment and exercise herself. She rode her scooter to the physical therapy facility and worked on the machines two hours every day.

After these sessions, Dare would drive her chair around town, visiting various stores and friends. She was independent and determined to do things on her own, wheeling herself down the streets and often riding on the side of roads and highways to avoid traffic. I remember getting phone calls several times at work from people in the community who reported seeing Dare crossing intersections and highways where she might be hit by cars. When I would confront her regarding those concerns, she would often say, "Those busy-bodies need to mind their own business and not be such tattle tails! If I'm hit by a car at least I am doing something fun and living my life!"

Dare's attitude and determination to make the best out of her condition continued with an outward smile and high spirit as she faced the challenges. I was amazed how she conducted herself and continued to show others that she was a strong and independent lady in her daily activities despite being limited. Whether or not internal fears were present, she wasn't going to show a negative attitude from the hardships she faced.

Dare:

I enjoyed working out on my own and did this for several months. After doing physical therapy for so many years, I sometimes felt I needed to take a break. Then I would stop for a few months before going back. As time went on, my ability to complete some of the exercises waned. I would tell myself, "Well, this is a progressive disease, and I am supposed to go down, down, down." However, I still kept plugging along, trying to escape that number "10" on the disability chart....death!

When I was able to ride my scooter I drove myself. And even when I got into a mobilized wheelchair, I used my left hand to drive around town. It was so much fun going around, meeting friends and traveling around. Some of Keith's co-workers bought me a cell phone and paid for the minutes, but I didn't use it much because I didn't want the phone ringing and people wanting to know my whereabouts. If I needed help, someone along the way would respond. I felt totally comfortable on my own, but whenever some nut from Keith's workplace said they were scared for me, I would respond by saying they needed to attend to their own business! I was capable of managing myself, and it was a wonderful feeling. Just because everyone else was scared for me didn't mean there was a valid reason for this. I paid attention and saved my own life twice by looking out for crazy drivers. Just because I was in a wheelchair, didn't mean I didn't have a brain!

One thing that did bother me about being in a

wheelchair, though, is when people would talk to Keith and avoid eye contact with me...as if I wasn't able to speak for myself. I am still a person!

Keith:

In the summer of 1999, therapeutic horseback riding became another recommended intervention. We never thought riding on the back of a horse would be of benefit. However, we learned that the movement of the horse would help Dare to improve her balance and core strength. I gave her support and encouraged her to try the intervention. We located a nurse who had started a program.

Dare participated in weekly sessions, but without control of her legs, was scared to ride. In order to mount the horse, I would push her wheelchair up a ramp until the horse was below us. Lifting her from the chair, we placed her sideways on the horse's back. While supporting her back, we held her leg and stretched it over the back of the horse. At one point in the process, she would be lying almost flat on the horse while we got her situated and sitting up. From that point, she would be led around the ring by volunteers as she adjusted to the rhythm.

While successful, she was always scared of falling off the horse. She didn't feel secure sitting on its back without the benefit of using her legs to grip the horse. She hated this activity but continued to face her fears in hopes of a positive outcome.

We laughed every week as we drove to the lesson. Dare prayed for rain! And if she heard thunder, she was excited because the sessions would be cancelled. I was proud of her determination and persistence. She continued with this intervention, usually held from May to September, for four seasons. I don't know if I can be convinced that it helped with her balance, but I do feel it gave her confidence to face further challenges with her illness.

Dare began using a manual wheelchair in 1998 when walking long distances. She was resistant at first, not wanting to be in a chair. However, I confronted her and stated that it wasn't fair to me when she couldn't join in walks or activities. She finally agreed to use a chair to make it easier to participate.

Even during the stress of an unknown future, we worked to keep life as normal and spent time as a family. I remember taking the family out to dinner. We would drive to the parking area, and I'd get the chair from the trunk and set it up. With the stiffness in her legs, she had an awful time getting out of the car, after which point I would escort her to the table. The kids would be with us, and quickly adjusted to the looks from customers as we arranged the chair under the table.

Dare:

I must admit, I did the horseback riding therapy... but I didn't love it. When I was a child, we had a very mean pony. It tried to knock me off by running under trees, branches, or clotheslines. It also took a big hunk out of my brother's back. It would paw the ground when it was getting ready to roll over and we had to jump off in a hurry. I also knew a little boy who was kicked in the head and killed. No wonder I had a preconceived notion that horses could be dangerous! The therapy horses were so much taller than the pony.

After my childhood experiences, I was nervous getting on a horse's back. But I went along with the plan. My first horse, Duke, was 26 years old and very gentle. However, I did get a little scared when they placed me on another horse, Bud, who unexpectedly took off up the hill after an apple.

I didn't want to be a quitter, but I cried more than once and would praise God every time it rained! At this point, I had control of the reins but not my legs. This wasn't the most fun I ever had, but I made it through.

CHAPTER 16

A BIRTHDAY CELEBRATION

Keith:

On Dare's 45th birthday, I arranged to have a surprise song played for her. I told Dare we were going to a meeting at our church to talk about how we could service the disabled. She went along, thinking this was to be a new ministry. When we arrived at the church, we were greeted by the music director, who was dressed in a black tuxedo. Dare asked him why he was so dressed up. He told her he had just performed at a wedding. She thought nothing of it as I secretly laughed.

We entered the church sanctuary, where the stage was lit with candles and flowers. There were a few friends sitting along with the minister. Soon the lights dimmed. The music director came out, sat at the piano, and announced to Dare that this song was for her. I had chosen the song,

"To Make you Feel my Love" by Garth Brooks, from the movie *Hope Floats*. n playing the piano and sang that song.

It was a surprise, and special night of celebration for both of us.

Dare:

I must admit that Keith pulled one over on me. He gave me balloons, roses, and Beanie Babies®, which I collected. It was a beautiful night, and one I will never forget.

CHAPTER 17

CELEBRATION OF INDEPENDENCE

Keith:

In 2000 we found a scooter in a thrift shop, which Dare could drive with one hand. We bought it, and this gave her a feeling of freedom and independence. She would take herself to physical therapy, working with a therapist to do her strength and range of motion exercises. After her workout, Dare drove herself across the busy highway and to downtown. She visited with friends at the Council on Aging thrift store, often buying items that she could give to others. After shopping there, she would go to a local restaurant, sit and visit with the wait staff, and linger till I was able to walk and meet her after work. We would have dinner, walk home, and then I would return to my place of employment to pick up my car. We just wanted to spend nice afternoons and evenings enjoying each other and trying to make the best out of our situation.

Some days, Dare asked me to drop her off at the mall. I would protest, saying that she had no way to travel home, but she said she didn't want to go home. She would shop, meet friends, talk to sales clerks, and spend the whole day at the mall. Dare could stay in one section of a store for hours at a time, looking at things and entertaining herself. At this time, she was still independent, able to feed herself and use her hands to drive her power chair.

She enjoyed having the freedom to be out of the house and functioning on her own. There was no stopping her adventures and times. She reminded me that with the progression of her illness, there would come a day when she wasn't able to be independent and she planned to make the best of the days that were given to her to enjoy. To her, each day she could be out and enjoy life was a celebration of independence. I didn't try to stop her wishes and would drop her off in the morning and pick her up after work.

Dare:

Those were the good old days. I enjoyed the time away from the isolation at home. It's like the time I went to Ireland by myself at age 20. It gave me such a feeling, being able to do things on my own again. I felt free and independent. Being able to have some independence gave me such an appreciation of freedom.

CHAPTER 18

SOLEMN NEWS

Keith:

On our visit to the MS center in Charlotte in July of 2000, Dr. Kemp wanted Dare to have another MRI to check on the progression of the illness. When we returned home, she completed the MRI at the local hospital. The results were sent to Dr. Ball, her primary physician, who then wanted Dare to come to his office to discuss the results. He didn't ask to have me present. The doctor said, "Dare, you need to get your affairs in order. You need to be ready to go at a moment's notice!" He further explained that she had a large lesion on the brain stem that could immediately stop her breathing.

Dare said, "When the Master Physician calls, I'll be ready. But in the meantime, I'm not going to spend my time cleaning out drawers and files, because when I die, Keith will call a dumpster and haul my things away."

At the same time, Dare was taken by surprise the doctor's approach delivering this new information. She felt that without her strong personality or outlook on life, a statement like, "you need to get your affairs in order immediately," could throw another person into a deep depression to the point of considering suicide. However, even when she was alone and heard this warning, she felt strong enough to place her trust in God.

Dare came to see me at the hospital and reported what Dr. Ball said. I was shocked and replied, "I want to take you to Harvard. I want to know that if you were to die immediately, I did everything I knew possible." She said, "Atlanta was affiliated with Harvard, and they would tell me if I needed to do something." In other words, Dare wasn't going to spend whatever time she had on this earth in a panic and chasing after answers that nobody knew!

Dare:

I was taken aback when Dr. Ball told me to have my affairs in order, and unsure how I should feel about this statement. Should I be more concerned about the possibility? Shouldn't we all be ready to go at a moment's notice? I said to him, "Well, my next-door neighbor had heart trouble at age forty and the community worried about her. She lived to be 96 years old and buried three husbands. I'm a believer that if there is life, there is hope. I further believe that God will see me through whatever life gives me. Whether I live or die, it is all in His hands. There is no reason to worry until that time."

When I left his office, I met a friend for lunch and asked her how she would react if her doctor told her the same thing. The friend hugged me and said, "Oh Dare, you get to be with Anna in heaven!" But I said, "I have a husband and two children on earth. When I die, I'll have eternity to be with those who have gone before me. I want to stay on earth for as long as I can to see my children and future grandchildren grow."

Part of me wondered if I needed to take his statements more seriously. But to me, life is an adventure. My philosophy is if you're going to live a long life, you need to learn to live with many losses.

CHAPTER 19

RESPIRATORY ILLNESS

Keith:

In 2000 I became sick with a respiratory problem and had to stay in bed. Dare had never seen me this sick, but she had no concerns about contracting my same illness.

Unfortunately, her immune system was weak and she did become sick, requiring hospitalization for five days with another 25 days in a rehabilitation center. During her time in the rehab center, we agreed to have Elizabeth take a car to school. On Labor Day weekend, Elizabeth was supposed to return home for a visit. She was scheduled to arrive by 5:30 p.m. but when the time came, she didn't show up. By 6:30, I was in a panic when I hadn't heard from her.

I began calling every hospital and law enforcement office between Hendersonvill   )ne. I was so frightened that she had had an acci   may have gone over the mountain. I stared out (dow in hopes of seeing her car lights as I called around. I thought to myself, "Not only is Dare in the hospital, now Elizabeth is nowhere to be found." This is an example of how intense I can be when it comes to the condition of my family.

Finally, at 8:45 p.m., she called to tell me she had been in a minor accident, but she hadn't had the cell service to call. She had to wait until the highway patrol arrived to take a report. I was so thankful to hear she was safe, but the fright of not hearing had me half crazy. I couldn't even visit Dare that evening, afraid to tell her that Elizabeth wasn't home yet, and concerned how she would receive any negative news in her condition.

CHAPTER 20

LIFE CONTINUES

Keith:

When Dare returned home in late September of 2000, she was placed on homebound status, with visits from a nurse to check on her vital signs and general health. One of the criteria for receiving homebound services was the stipulation that the patient remain home, only leaving the house for medical appointments, church, or to have hair done. If she didn't stay home she would be dismissed from services. At the time of Dare's discharge from the rehabilitation center, she met the homebound requirements. She didn't have the energy to care for herself.

It took a number of months for Dare to regain health. When she began feeling better and recovered her strength, she told the home health agency to discontinue services. She planned to leave the house, which was not allowed. Dare said she was leaving anyway, and on her scooter to boot! She felt too confined and wasn't willing to remain home.

Later in the spring, after Dare's recovery, we told Dr. Kemp about Dare's discussion with Dr. Ball about being "ready to go at a moment's notice." Dr. Kemp said the lesion on the brain stem had actually been there for some time, but was inactive. He didn't feel Dare was in immediate danger. While this certainly relieved my fear, I couldn't help but think about the additional stress those statements had placed on us. We returned home feeling grateful and continued living the best we could under the circumstances.

In 2002 our son, who was a senior in high school, played baseball and we enjoyed watching his activity. One evening the team had a recognition night for the seniors. They had the mothers come onto the field to meet their sons, who then gave them a flower. Dare was rather embarrassed because she had to drive her scooter onto the field in front of others. That was something Dare never liked to do…walk in front of others.

This night was no exception. She had to drive down the sideline to find an opening onto the field. By the time she made it out, others were waiting. I think she became so nervous she had a hard time moving her chair. However, Andrew didn't mind having to wait for her, and the crowd seemed to understand. But for Dare it was another reminder that she was different. When she met Andrew, his flower had a broken stem. Dare made the comment, "A broken flower for a broken mom," and laughed as usual. When nervous and under stress, Dare makes wild statements.

It wasn't too long after that we had an opportunity to purchase a couple more scooters. I'm not sure why we had a total of three, but one afternoon Dare, Andrew, and another friend had a parade going to town, each one driving a scooter across the highway, past the high school, and into town to have lunch. Andrew and his friend rode their scooters into the restaurant to eat with Dare. The stares and laughs they got that day were worth the trip.

On another occasion Dare and her cousin, Marsha, rode the scooters to a thrift store. Marsha bought a hat that looked like Minnie Pearl and drove to the courthouse. When the wind blew her hat off, Marsha got off her scooter and ran after it. Folks laughed, thinking she also had to use a handicapped scooter to get around town! Dare's thought was, "If you can't beat 'em, you might as well join 'em."

In the spring of 2001, we bought our first handicapped van with a ramp. The ramp rattled as we rode down the road, but it was so convenient to have a vehicle that enabled us to use a motorized power chair for transport. We also purchased hand controls to put on the steering wheel so Dare could drive and apply brakes via hand devices. One of her last long-distance driving trips was when she and daughter Elizabeth drove to see her parents. Dare drove about 100 out of the 200 miles using the hand control, then had Elizabeth finish the drive when she became tired.

Finally, on Dare's 50th birthday in 2004, she decided to hand in her driver's license instead of renewing, telling the instructor, "Happy Birthday to me!" She felt it was getting harder to operate the car and she didn't feel safe behind the steering wheel. She was concerned about making the transfer from chair to chair and operating the hand controls to apply the brake. The instructor asked if she wanted to try and renew but Dare said she didn't feel it was worth the worry. She did ask if she could still come back should she change her mind. He assured her that she could.

This has made me the primary driver for the past 17 years for our travel. It includes taking Dare to her appointments, shopping, outings, and special events...

another role added to the caretaker's list.

During the early years of the illness, Dare was still able to use her hands and could carry on the daily activities of dressing, hair washing, and cooking. She pushed herself to maintain as much energy as possible to give attention to her children's activities, school functions, and sporting events. At one such sporting event our daughter, Elizabeth, hit the ball and collided with another girl while playing in a high school soccer game. This resulted in a mouth injury needing medical attention. Dare and I were in the stands when we saw the accident. Dare tried to come down to the field, but under the anxiety of the moment had difficulty walking. I told her that by the time she made it to the field, Elizabeth would bleed to death! We agreed I would escort Elizabeth to the hospital while another friend would drive Dare.

We adjusted to the various changes occurring as the illness progressed, never knowing when the next adventure was headed our way. One such adventure took place when my father decided to have a family reunion at the Grove Park Inn in Asheville, an exceptionally fine resort inn and host to many celebrities over the years. Dad's health was failing, but he had inherited a sum of money and therefore wanted to have this reunion before he died. He invited his brother from Texas and another brother from

Florida, along with spouses, children, and grandchildren.

Dare and I prepared that night for this very formal dinner. However, on the way over, our old van broke down on the side of the road. Luckily, I had my cell phone and called my brother to rescue us. I wasn't sure what happened to our car, but by the time we made it to the party, we were sweating and looked like mountain hillbillies! What's even worse, the van broke down again on the way home, only this time we had family members following us. I transported Dare to another vehicle and left her chair in the van until we could service it the next day. Luckily, I had a manual wheelchair to utilize at home.

We continued to patch up the car for several more years until some friends told us of a couple from Florida who had a used van. The wife had died and the husband wanted to sell. These friends went to Florida and brought the car back to us. It felt so much better having a reliable van for travel. It was especially important to have decent transportation for long trips when we had to transport Dare with her chair and other equipment.

In 2010 we were referred to a "seating assessment clinic" to measure Dare for an enhanced power chair. Medicare assisted with some of the cost, although we still paid $2,500 for the order. This chair not only allowed Dare to drive with her hand but allowed her to move the seat up and down to reposition herself. This was the very first time we realized she would basically be confined to a power chair for all her movement and activities.

Dare remained stable until 2011, when she started losing function in her hands. In the beginning of her illness, we were told that her upper extremities would more than likely not be affected. However, she began noticing weakness and great difficulty writing with her right hand. In the coming months, she could no longer use her right hand but was still able to drive her wheelchair with her left hand to go to town, appointments, and shopping. She learned to use her left hand using occupational therapy hand exercises, which also taught her to pick up rocks, place stamps on envelopes, and write.

Occupational therapy helped some, but soon weakness began in her left hand and Dare lost the ability to use both. With losing her ability to walk or use her hands, Dare has had to rely on me for all daily living activities: dressing, toileting, and personal care.

In the mornings, I lift her out of bed and transfer her to a bedside toilet. I hold her up while she uses the toilet, wipe her behind, and lift her back into her wheelchair. I then dress her, putting on her bra, shirt, and skirt (she dresses in skirts because she cannot stand for me to put on pants and pull them up). After she's initially seated in her wheelchair, I hold her while putting the back of the chair down so I can pull her the rest of the way into the chair. After settling her fully in the chair, I cook breakfast and then sit next to her while I feed her.

After breakfast, she usually likes to read. However, without the ability to turn pages in books or magazines, I turn each page and position the book against a pillow so she has access to read. She needs to reposition herself several times an hour, and I spend time moving the chair into various positions to take some of the pressure off her back and hips. When using the telephone, I dial the number and place the phone in a position for her to speak. The phone is not able to disconnect calls, so I remain available to hang up after each call.

We go through basically the same routine for lunch and dinner, with me preparing and feeding meals to her. At lunch, I give medications with fluid so she can swallow each tablet. After supper, we spend time undressing, toileting, lifting into a chair/bed, covering, and positioning her for relaxation.

One of the side effects of being in a power chair 24/7 is skin breakdown on the pressure points of her butt from not being able to move. Fortunately, Dare still has feeling in her limbs and can tell when a skin breakdown is occurring. Without this sensation, a skin breakdown could evolve to the point of severe infection, which then leads to additional, major complications. This type of breakdown continues to occur, requiring my help and the use of pain patches for wound dressing and healing. We had home health orders for a nurse to provide wound care. Thus far, we've been able to address wound care needs with basic pain patches and medications.

In the evenings, Dare and I try to find humor and ways to work around our losses to cope with the stresses and changes in our life. One activity we miss is dancing because it's no longer possible to hold her in my arms. We used to go to a summer music concert where they had bands playing beach and soul music. The crowd would sit on lawn chairs and on the ground. Often, people would dance to the music. To enjoy the event, I would stand her up in my arms and we would sway to the music. However, after several seasons, she could no longer stand long enough to be comfortable, and I had a hard time holding her up. Then I tried to dance with her sitting in her power chair. We would get lots of stares, but I really didn't mind; I've always loved to dance. We find a way to enjoy the music, even if it requires the movement of her chair and my being tangled in the wheels!

On a visit to Dr. Kemp in 2013, I told him of Dare's decline with her hands a̲ ̲ ̲ ̲ ̲ ̲ to speak with him. Dare stated she didn't wish ̲ ̲ ̲ ̲ rt of this conversation, so Dr. Kemp agreed to ̲ ̲ ̲ ̲ ̲ ̲ private. When I sat down with him, he looked at me and said, "I know what you want to discuss. You want to know what the future looks like."

While he couldn't give me a timeline for the progression of her decline, he did state that in many similar cases he often begins seeing an effect on major organs of the body impacting things such as eating and breathing. There can be the need for a ventilator to assist in breathing. There is the possibility of losing bladder and bowel control. At this point, hard decisions have to be made regarding feeding tubes, ventilators, and end-of-life decisions. Again, he tried to be hopeful but also felt he needed to be honest about possible issues.

One of the most difficult parts of this illness is watching the deterioration of the person I love, and worrying about the children's reactions and feelings toward their mother. Currently, both children appear to be dealing with her limitations. They don't want to talk about any negative feelings. It's almost like sitting in the living room with an elephant. I know they are concerned, close, and loving. But they don't want to acknowledge future progression.

CHAPTER 21

ANOTHER DIAGNOSIS

Keith:

June 25, 2019 was the morning of my 68th birthday. It was also the day Dare was referred to the cancer center for assessment of some abnormal blood results. She had elevated platelets, which placed her at a higher risk of stroke. After several tests, it was determined that she had a blood disorder known as essential thrombocythemia (ET), a "cousin" to leukemia. This blood disorder is classified as a type of cancer. However, Dr. Ray, our oncologist, stated this could be treated with an oral chemotherapy medication. He felt that once it was under control, she could continue a "normal" life expectancy but may have to remain on an oral type of chemo to maintain platelet levels.

I thought, "How can this be happening? Not only do we live with a crippling disease, but now we must face another issue. How much more can we endure?"

The diagnosis was a complete surprise to the both of us. Several of her family members have had similar blood disorders, with some leading to higher risk of stroke. Dr. Ray started Dare on chemotherapy by taking a daily tablet which required regular blood draws to check her platelet levels.

Dare's veins have been ruined after the previous chemotherapy treatment and IV steroids for the MS. After several visits to withdraw blood, the nurses sometimes had to insert the needles several times to get blood flow. With this difficulty, Dr. Ray recommended a port to facilitate the monthly blood draws. We discussed this option and Dare underwent a procedure to insert a port in November 2019. We now make monthly trips to flush the port, and visit Dr. Ray every three months for blood tests. We hope those visits will become less frequent.

After eleven visits, the levels looked good and there was no need to increase medication. But he still wanted us to continue the protocol of monthly port flushes and six-month consults. If the platelet counts increase, we will need to increase the chemotherapy. We learned from blood levels that she also needs to increase her levels of Vitamin D.

We recently followed up with him and learned that Dare's platelet levels increased slightly over the past six months. Therefore, he increased her chemotherapy medication from nine pills a week to ten. We're due to return in six months.

Dare stays in a dehydrated state much of the time because increased fluid intake leads to an increased need to urinate, which then requires using the toilet. Currently she tries to limit that undertaking to two times a day because the task of toileting is significant in its complexity. It requires transferring her from chair to bedside toilet, wiping, and transferring back to the middle of the chair. From there, one needs to pull her back the rest of the way into her chair, adjust her legs, and replace her pillows for core strength optimization.

When transferring, the biggest concerns are the risk of losing balance and the risk of a fall, both for Dare and the person assisting. We place the toilet and chair close together to minimize this risk. In an attempt to minimize it further, we purchased a $7,000 lift to assist in transfers, which uses a sling tied around her and mechanisms to lift and lower her. The lift is supposed to minimize the chances of a fall while making it safer for those assisting her. However, the lift itself results in additional complications: the time it takes to place the sling around her, attaching it to the lift, then raising and lowering it to hit the "mark" before reversing the process to place her back in the chair.

I have found it quicker (not safer) to transfer with my arms around her body and lifting her with my strength. However, this is not the most secure and does create additional risk to my back, in addition to increasing the risk of a fall. It was our hope that the lift could be used when traveling, and that it could be used in someone else's home so they could assist her while I returned home for a respite. This would give her more frequent outside visits, especially to her parents. However, after being assured the lift could be taken apart for travel, we discovered it was very difficult to place in the car and re-assemble due to its size. We also discovered that the apparatus is so big there is no room in the home for setting it up! In hindsight, we should have purchased a much smaller lift, one that could be moved and transferred with less complication. I'm not sure why this particular model was purchased other than we lacked the experience to realize the trouble it would create.

Due to the recent Covid-19 virus, we've needed to take all the additional precautions required by the pandemic: following the guidelines of mask wearing, social distancing, hand washing, and avoiding contact with others. Dare has taken this warning very seriously, and we've elected not to have others in our home nor to attend activities outside the home (like our church services). Her medical condition is serious enough that she is at risk for contracting the disease. In fact, there's been changes at the cancer center for Dare and other patients. The regimen for flushing the port is now extended to every three months with office visits every six months. There is less risk with fewer visits.

Dare:

I was completely caught off guard when diagnosed with the blood cancer. I hadn't been feeling bad. The three months prior to the test, we were on a special diet (Paleo autoimmune protocol) that had us eating only completely healthy foods. We'd been on this diet for 100 days. So imagine my surprise when my bloodwork had highs and lows. We repeated the bloodwork five weeks later, and it wasn't better. We were referred to the oncologist, Dr. Ray, at the cancer center.

I went, thinking that I probably had something wrong with my blood that co‎ ‎sily treated. When he used the word "cance‎ ‎aken aback. I thought, "You have got to be ‎......‎. It didn't seem to hit me right away. However, over the next few days, I absorbed the impact and have since adjusted to the diagnosis. As one person told me, "Girl, you've got this! After all, you've dealt with MS!"

Looking back on previous blood test results, the oncologist felt this might have started around 2015, and I think he might be right. He also told me he would rather have this cancer than other types of cancer. I asked, "So you would rather have this than prostate cancer?" He said, "Yes, I would. People can live ten or more years with this type of cancer." I did know a man at our church who had the same type of cancer for 26 years before passing away with acute leukemia.

I have survived many other things before this blood cancer. I think that, out of all the things I have endured, the cancer is not the worst. I am 67 years old and have had a good life. I have grown children and beautiful grandchildren. If my life ended now, I would have survived while enjoying my time.

CHAPTER 22

CHALLENGES AND FRUSTRATIONS FACED

Keith:

I never thought I would be in this situation. When I first heard that my wife was diagnosed with MS, I thought I would be able to care for her. I never realized how difficult the role of caretaker could be, nor how it would affect our relationship. This is not to say it's been all bad, but it comes with the realization that the marriage has changed profoundly.

One of my major challenges I have is admitting there is a difference in the balance of duties and responsibilities in our relationship. There used to be a sharing of needs in our relationship. Now it is a challenge to find other ways, resources, or people to meet those needs. And it takes endless planning, preparing, asking, and admitting to the struggle.

While we still have much for which we are grateful, there are times I find myself in grief over what could have been. I must remind myself of the illness's huge impact on our lives...and that it's not the person, but the illness which is to blame. It can be overwhelming to live up to the expectations of caregiving and providing for the basic needs of someone else on a daily basis. It becomes a challenge when I'm not only trying to accomplish my own daily functions, but those of my partner as well. When the stress becomes too much, I often find my emotions becoming raw and I overreact. Those interactions then lead to feelings of guilt. While I realize it's a normal reaction to stress and pressure, negative energy can become the norm in meeting the demands of the caretaking role.

One might think that taking care of each other is just a basic part of the "for better or worse, in sickness and health" vows of marriage, the commitment we make. But when this commitment becomes a day-in and day-out routine, it's a challenge. It takes a lot of energy to attend to another when all you want is to just take care of yourself.

There are challenges faced for the disabled and caregiver in the day-to-day routine. Due to Dare's lack of mobility, she is not able to sleep in a regular bed. She is not able to roll over, move her legs, or wiggle her feet. When she's in bed, she stays in one position and that becomes too uncomfortable for sleep. So she often stays in her power chair at night, where she can use a device called a "head ray" which allows her to move up and down, and elevate feet. While this has been better, it forces her to stay in her chair 24/7. This, in turn, creates problems with skin breakdown and pressure wounds requiring medical intervention.

Dare still has sensation and feeling in all her extremities, and it's a blessing in many ways. If she couldn't feel, wounds would go unnoticed and the possibility of infection (and death) from sepsis would increase. It's a negative in that Dare experiences aspects of MS that are quite painful.

One of these is known as "Lhermitte's sign," which is a sudden sensation of electric shock that runs from the neck to the spine and legs or arms. She often has these painful spasms from her right shoulder going down the legs. When these occur, she's in severe pain for about 15 seconds before they subside, and says it feels like her legs are on fire. At other times, she may feel episodes of pain in her knees and legs, possible symptoms of MS.

During these episodes she yells and asks for a massage to alleviate the pain. We're about to try a masseuse, who is coming to the home to assist in muscle release and relaxation, to see if it helps.

Other challenges exist for which we've not been prepared.

For example, we purchased membership with AAA as protection in the event of car trouble. One time our car broke down and I called them, explaining that my wife was totally disabled. They were very responsive to my car needs with their assistance but could not transport the car with my wife inside. I explained that it wasn't possible to get her into a regular car without difficulty. Not only was she not able to use her legs to make a safe transfer, but she would have no access to her power chair. And I couldn't leave her on the side of the road! But they were firm: this was a liability issue, and the insurance (or law) would not allow them to move the car with her inside.

I wasn't aware of any transfer service that could transport her and accommodate her chair. I called our van emergency number; they could send a van, but the cost was over $100 an hour and would start at the time of the call. I then called an ambulance and was told it would be over $400 to transport her. I finally called a friend whose car had a large back seat, and they came to the rescue. We still had to move her from my higher car seat to the lower vehicle. And we also had to leave the power chair in the van to be transported with the tow truck. But at least we had a regular wheelchair at home for mobility.

This experience raised the concern that if we had car trouble while traveling further from home, how could we accommodate her disability? We would either be stuck on the side of the road or need to utilize an expensive alternative. I thought of keeping a regular, fold-down wheelchair in the car for an event where I needed to move her to another car. In which case I would again need to leave our expensive, 500-pound power chair behind and hope it was still there when the car was returned to us.

Other issues are more humorous and/or embarrassing. There is a bolt under her chair designed to lock the chair into the van floor. However, this bolt easily catches anything in its path, including high rugs and ledges. Rugs then catch and twist underneath the chair.

We were attending a wedding in a very formal inn. As we entered the front lobby, the chair became hooked on an oriental rug, which then wrapped around the bolt. Luckily, I did not have to cut the rug loose, but it took over 20 minutes to unwrap. I've since learned to be more aware of rugs into entrance areas of restaurants. However, I don't always judge correctly and have had several close calls. What a challenge just to get something to eat!

Just recently, Dare and I were going into a restaurant and the waiter was escorting us to a suitable table. There was a partition separating the lobby from the dining area. I tried to drive the power chair while also aiming for the table. It was a tight area, and I ran into the partition. There was a loud sound, and the petition began to tip. Luckily, both the waiter and I were fast enough to catch the partition before it fell over. But everyone in the dining area looked up, and their eyes followed us to our table. I told Dare I was so embarrassed I wanted to go to the bathroom and hide! Again, what a challenge!

It's amazing that, for all the handicapped accessibility laws on the books, there are many places still not truly accessible. We've become very aware of the need to check accommodations before visiting a venue. We have a favorite restaurant, located in a basement, which has service on the sidewalk above. But this means we have to fight flies, gnats, and other bugs if we try to eat at this establishment.

Many healthcare facilities have poor access for the handicapped. I often have a challenge trying to open doors while also negotiating her chair...a very basic oversight for a medical institution! You'd think a medical facility would be more aware.

We've had challenges with city streets, sidewalks, and pavement. We've had to maneuver around telephone poles in the middle of the sidewalk and navigate broken concrete. Often there are uneven walks, resulting in painfully bumpy rides which aggravate wounds and sores. In fact, I once tripped on an uneven sidewalk, falling and breaking my glasses, receiving cuts and a black eye!

When we first moved into our apartment building, the spot assigned to our car didn't have a handicapped-accessible ramp. There was instead a four-inch curb and an elevated threshold preventing entrance to the building. I purchased threshold ramps which gave us access over the curb and placed another ramp on the steps leading to the main sidewalk. The homeowner's association apparently took pictures of this and sent our landlady a letter demanding everything allowing us access be removed. They felt if they made accommodations for one tenant, they would have to make accommodations for every disabled tenant. They felt that because the building was built before handicapped-accessible laws were in place, they were grandfathered in and therefore didn't have to make changes. In fact, one neighbor told me if we weren't satisfied with the facility, we should move.

I reviewed all the handicapped laws, took pictures of the areas where we were challenged, and threatened to take legal action. After much discussion between their members and attorneys, a resolution was agreed upon allowing accommodations that were satisfactory to our needs. One neighbor kindly offered to change her parking space to allow us better access for our car ramp. This neighbor showed compassion and understanding, but overall, it wasn't the greatest welcome to a new home.

It certainly fuels the challenge to continue the fight for change. People who fail in their awareness or compassion to the disabled don't realize the day-to-day impediments these citizens face until they are directly involved themselves. Many people have been incredibly supportive and helpful in meeting our needs when we're faced with obstacles. We often hear statements like, "We never thought about this issue before." So while not easy, in some ways our challenges provide an unexpected opportunity to educate others.

We have equipment that includes wheelchairs, canes, walkers, a lift chair and bed, a bedside toilet, a transfer lift, a Hoyer lift, and vans. Every five years, Medicare allows us to replace our power wheelchair. When ordering or buying these items from merchants, there are times the salesperson will ask me, "What does she want?" as if her disability and need for a wheelchair makes her incapable of responding. I often reply, "She's not ignorant and she can talk. Believe me, she has a mouth!"

The caregiving role has an impact on marriage, changing the balance in a marriage as caretaking needs manifest. While there is a bond, there is now also an imbalance. The partnership changes regardless of the love. There is a change in the level of intimacy. There are questions of trust, abandonment, and fear of the unknown.

Both parties are faced with loss. And make no mistake, there is a loss of independence for both parties. The disabled spouse relies on the caregiver for most of their needs, placing extra burden and responsibility on one person. As the impact on the marriage increases, there is an ongoing need to openly discuss losses and changes. This is not easy to accept; but is attainable.

Dare:

The Lhermitte's sign spasm episodes have occurred more over the past few months, which I feel is a symptom of MS progression. When I have them, they start in my neck and shoulder and move down to my legs. It feels as though my legs are on fire, an overwhelming sensation which makes me distraught. The spasms last for about 15 to 20 seconds, and sometimes the pain is so severe that I have to call to Keith to help me.

When I'm awakened by these painful spasms in the morning, I try to remain calm so Keith can have his morning coffee before I ask for his help. But nighttime is when I experience the most pain and discomfort, and I need to wake him. He massages, lifts, and repositions my legs until I find relief from the burning. All the while I feel guilty and sad that I've had to wake him.

It's when in pain like this from MS that I feel the most discouraged and disappointed. I'm not a particularly good pain warrior. During these episodes, I sometimes say, "I can't take it anymore." Keith replies, "You don't have a choice." I can handle the losses and the normal progressions. I have learned to handle most of the challenges. But I feel very weak when it comes to pain. I pray for relief. I don't want to live with medications.

CHAPTER 23

FEELINGS AND CONFLICTS

Keith:

Today I am sitting under the buckeye tree seeking shade from the fall sunshine. The breeze is warm and the sky is a brilliant blue. My mind races with many thoughts. I find myself alone, thinking of my life's journey over the past years as my wife's primary caretaker. Please understand that I share my experience in hope of providing a truthful and honest look at the role of so many in my position.

As I mentioned earlier, love is a four-letter word that has a broad meaning. I want to start by saying I've had a good relationship with my wife over the years of our marriage, and I love her. But caretaking isn't easy and there are so many conflicting emotions attached to it. I deal with frustration and anger as a result of her illness. (And to be clear – it's the illness that has created the resentment, pain, and anger, not the person.)

When she was first diagnosed, I told myself I was strong enough to handle whatever the illness gave us. I strived for perfection and gave the appearance that caretaking could be accomplished with little effort on my part. I had a family I loved and a wife who gave me meaning and purpose. We had our times of struggle and disagreements during those first years, but underneath them was commitment and love.

I continue with that commitment, although with a different meaning of love. For me, my love has deepened as I've continued to stay close to her side. I have not abandoned her, like so many others put in a similar position. I'm not being judgmental toward those who decide to leave their loved one. I believe tough decisions must be made either way, and one must do what's best for all concerned. I'm just saying that for me, it is what it is, and I will do what I need to do no matter the perceptions or values of others.

Dare told me that she still "loves me" as she always did. But she feels my definition of love has changed. Things do change to some extent. I feel I have changed and grown. I've become stronger as a person and continue to provide caregiving duties despite times I would prefer to run away. Is that love?

When one is in their 20s and takes a vow of marriage, one does it without knowing what that future might bring. Love is commitment, dedication, loyalty, responsibility, and service...especially to one that has become totally disabled.

Dare was initially able to do many things independently in the early years of her illness. For example, she was able to dress, use the bathroom, and bathe herself. She was able to feed herself and drive a car with hand controls. She was able to use her hands to drive a scooter without help. She could help with washing clothes, cooking, cleaning house, and taking care of laundry. She could scratch her nose, comb her hair, and apply makeup to her face. As her illness progressed, she lost her ability to do these activities and started relying on me...not only to take on personal caretaking, but household chores and many of the necessary activities of daily living. (If I sound resentful or angry, it's accurate, again not toward my wife but toward what this illness has done to our relationship.)

Those who do not live in the situation cannot fully understand this role. For example, last night we were leaving one of our favorite sandwich shops when the infamous locking bolt under the power chair got caught on the rug at the restaurant. The rug wrapped itself under the wheels and we became stuck, unable to go forward or backward. This is one of those times where I become embarrassed, frustrated, angry, and tired from the hassle that this illness has created.

There are so many times I've tried to put on a positive face when out in public, when in reality I've wanted to run away. Instead, I'm on the floor of the restaurant trying to untangle the rug. The chair has taken out many rugs! When this happened at Pizza Hut, it took the manager and cook forty-five minutes to cut the rug loose.

Most recently, Dare and I attended the first wrestling match of our grandson, Gavin. When we arrived at the event, Dare's seat belt got tangled underneath the wheel of her chair. I had to go to the passenger side of the car to expand the belt in order to release her. However, the belt would not expand, and I was on the floor of the van trying to gain some slack in the belt to move her chair back. After moving the chair back and forth in the front seat, I was finally able to get the belt off the wheel.

Another frustration for me centers around meals. I'm not a great cook, nor do I find myself interested in learning. I can skip meals or eat light, enjoy a variety and quantity of food. I become frustrated trying to fix Dare something to eat because I really don't enjoy making meals.

These are just a few examples of the frustrations that come with certain tasks. There are many moments I don't want the caretaking responsibility. Neither does she want to be in the position in which she finds herself. She never wanted to be dependent on anyone else to meet her needs or entertain her.

Her disease progression has caused me to realize her needs require more care than any one person can give. I deal with guilt, stress, anger, resentment, lack of energy, and lack of motivation. I ask myself how I can continue to meet all her needs and stay positive at the same time. I share this fact in order to be honest and open…and to ask forgiveness in not being all she needs.

We can no long travel with spontaneity, not when it includes packing a bedside toilet or needing to question whether or not every single place we go is handicapped accessible. As I've said, we are no longer able to dance, the one activity I strongly miss (although I get lots of looks at concerts when I try to dance with her wheelchair; I don't have that one down completely). We cannot hold hands as we once did. Physical intimacy has changed, although we still have those special moments of eye contact and knowing what each is thinking or wishing. Of course, she has her own anger and grief toward the illness. Many times, she expresses a desire to walk again or to simply have the ability to use one hand to do many of the daily routines for her own care. However, in the positive and loving part of our relationship, she deals with her situation with the most gracious and positive attitude. She has such a warm smile, strong faith, a love of family, a love of our marriage.

While I share many of her positive attributes, I must express how hard this is for both of us if I am to be honest about my emotions. We deal with our losses – in their distinct forms – together. But there are times my frustration becomes hard to control and I say negative things that leave me feeling guilt and remorse. However, she keeps forgiving me, knowing these outbursts are my expression of frustration. Regardless, it's still not right and I am trying to work on better and more productive ways to express my feelings while trying to give her care at home.

We've discussed the possibility of placement in a nursing facility. I realize that I'm getting older and less able to provide for her physical needs, and it may reach a point where we need nursing home placement. However, I've dealt with many nursing homes in my career of hospital case management and discharge planning. I know very well the care – or lack of care – patients can receive. So many lack the staff to provide adequate care. Often, a patient may have to wait long periods of time to receive the attention they need.

Dare feels she isn't ready to accept nursing home placement; she feels she gets the best care at home with my help. She is more likely to accept placement in a facility if I go with her! However, I'm not willing to pay the price for nursing home care if I'm the one who ends up doing much of it at the facility.

At one time, we had a lady (who had previously worked for Dare) move into the house to help. She'd been forced to move out of her apartment and needed a place to live, and we needed extra help with day-to-day activities. She had two dogs that she wanted to bring with her, so we agreed to it provided the dogs stayed upstairs so as not to bother Dare's cat.

For the first two months, this arrangement seemed to benefit both parties. However, the relationship soon began to change, and the lady began taking advantage of our situation. She allowed her dogs full access to the house. Her former partner visited more than we liked and smoked when he was there (although we asked him not to, due to Dare's allergies). We never felt we had privacy; she was always around us during the day.

While we initially thought we could be helpful to each other, the relationship soured and we finally asked her to move. She was incredibly angry with us, and it took us some time to explain the situation. We've since debated about trying to have someone live with us again. But the thought of giving up our privacy again leaves us leery of getting into another situation.

In addition to the logistical considerations of in-home help, we realize that cost is of extreme concern. Most qualified help requires a minimum of three to four hours per day, with a charge of $20 dollars per hour.

We know that circumstances may force us to eventually change our minds. While shared responsibility and additional assistance are the positive aspect of in-home care, we also need to consider what's best for our relationship. I do think that hiring help would be advantageous to reduce stress and the risk of injury.

Dare:

While I am not under the buckeye tree with Keith at the moment, I, too, find it frustrating to navigate the complexity of our situation. Since Keith and I were both public servants, we don't have an excess of monetary resources. Keith has social security benefits and a 401(k) plan. I have social security benefits and a partial pension. At the time I did chemotherapy, I was given the option to pay $1,000 and receive a full pension (I was eligible because of my age and number of years I taught). I had to sign papers to accept or decline the offer.

At that time, I wasn't worried about the future; I was so sick from chemo and the MS I didn't know if I would survive. And regardless of whether there was a future or not, we didn't have the $1,000. They say hindsight is 20/20, and we could certainly use that full pension now. As time goes on and we must consider in-home care, it will be difficult to have adequate resources to hire the extra help. We'll have to cross that bridge when we come to it.

In the beginning, Keith and I both thought I had the relapsing/remitting form of MS, and that I would be in remission from time to time. It was a surprise to see how quickly my health declined after the diagnosis in November of 1995. I now realize I probably had MS much earlier than that. When I take this into consideration, I had many happy years without an inkling that I had this illness.

Early on, Keith and I discussed the fact that if I had cancer, he would only need to be a super hero for a short period of time, and then it would be over. With MS it could be a ___ ___ ___ nger time than cancer. We were both optimi___ ___ ___ we could handle the disease. But now it's ___ ___ ___ ugher as the disease progresses and we get older.

Now, everything we do takes more planning and effort. Even when someone says a certain place is "accessible," it's not always as accessible as they think. There are many degrees of "accessible;" even if there is only one step up, my wheelchair cannot make the jump. Also, I cannot always know how I'm going to feel on the day of a planned activity.

It's a challenge, and I feel badly that my disease has affected Keith's life in such a drastic manner. Keith is a person with a big heart. He cares very deeply and goes beyond and above in what he does. Sometimes I think of what we would be doing if we hadn't been afflicted with this illness. I still think most things are doable – and I'd like to think we are up to the challenge – but sometimes I wonder. Everything requires so much more planning and patience than we sometimes have. Everything requires daily dependence upon my faith and Keith's effort to get through it. As I like to say, "It's not easy; it takes grit and grease to make it through."

CHAPTER 24

SIBLING CONCERNS

Keith:

One area of conflict has come from my siblings, who've expressed concern for my health realizing the work I do in my caregiving role. They've advocated placement in a nursing home, where Dare's care would be shared by a staff of people and I could visit and take her on daily outings. They don't understand the financial pressures of its cost, nor the quality-of-life issues present in nursing homes. While I realize they are frustrated and concerned with the situation, Dare feels that they are trying to "put her away."

And of course, that puts me in the middle. I honestly believe my siblings have the best of intentions and care about Dare. They see the struggles we have both endured with the illness.

Life itself has day-to-day stressors and takes effort meeting its daily demands. But when one is in a relationship with this much history and connection, it's hard just to think of oneself. Yes, I initially felt that a nursing home placement would be ideal for me and reduce the energy expended on care. However (as I ask my family), what does placement do to the individual? I know Dare is the type of person who would adjust and make friends wherever she might be, but to think of her spending her remaining time in a nursing facility, where she may not be given immediate attention to her needs, is more than I can currently tolerate.

One of my brothers has the attitude of "if not happy, find another." As a result, he's been involved in several marriages or relationships. I cannot imagine him taking on a role of caregiver to the extent I have. Put in the same position, I believe he would utilize the option of placement.

My second brother, who lives out of state, has been the most supportive of me. He does worry about my health and especially about the future as I age and Dare progressively declines. He provides me with support by keeping in touch with phone calls and listening to my struggles, frustrations, and conflicts. I know he has my interest at heart. Yet I still have to explain that, while my needs may not always be met, I have an obligation and commitment to do what I can to provide for Dare.

My sister, Kathy, is the one who introduced me to Dare. She lives close by and has been of assistance. She was also my mother's caregiver before her death, which helped reduce my worries and concerns at that time about not attending to my mother's needs along with my responsibility for Dare. Mom lived in an assisted living or nursing home for 12 years after my father's death.

I worked at the hospital but parked my car in the apartment complex where my mother lived, which was across the road from the hospital. Each morning as I drove to work, she would stand at the window, incredibly sad-looking and depressed after my father died. She finally had a breakdown and ended up in the mental health unit due to depression and anxiety. After her discharge, we felt she wasn't strong enough to maintain independent living. So my sister and I placed her in a facility where she would get help and attention for her needs.

My sister went every day to add to my mother's care, take her on outings, and shop for her. She will never know how much I appreciated her help with that; I already had so much responsibility at home caring for Dare, attending to the children's needs, and working a full-time job. It was such a relief having Kathy take on the caregiving role for Mom during the 12 years she lived in those facilities. She feels helpless now that she can't do more for me, but I appreciate all that she did caring for Mom.

I have a long history with Dare, and a commitment to my children. My life is not just about my needs or happiness. Although the role can be challenging, the devotion is strong. It's nice to have the concern of family members, but they don't know how our relationship has enriched my life regardless of caregiving needs or issues.

Dare:

I would not wish this illness on anyone. It is a struggle every day, and a constant reminder that I have to depend on others. I was always independent and never wanted to depend on others for my wellbeing, especially to live in this situation. When I married Keith, I thought I would be the caregiver to him and to our parents as they aged. Life doesn't always turn out the way we anticipate.

My feelings have been hurt the times I've heard the things Keith's family have said about "putting me away" in a nursing home. I have spent time in a nursing facility for rehabilitation after being hospitalized with a respiratory infection. On two occasions I also stayed in another nursing facility while Keith took a respite break.

Personally, I would prefer to stay in my home and hire extra help from an agency, which we've done as we've been able to afford. I don't need someone with me all the time, but to come for tasks such as feeding and toileting needs. Utilizing my head ray to move the chair, I've been able to stay home alone so Keith can be gone for several hours at a time. If he isn't able to be home by bedtime, I have a friend willing to assist in my care using a hoyer lift. I have a couple of friends who come over to walk me to town, have lunch, and socialize as well.

Presently my toileting needs can be met twice a day, once in the morning and again in the evening. I'm fortunate I don't need to be potted or fed more than that. I'm no longer able to stand on my feet and pivot to the chair for toileting needs, so Keith usually picks me up out of the chair and moves me without the use of a lift because he says it's faster. He's been told this isn't best for his back, but he insists that, so long as he has the ability, he prefers this method. We've had some falls, but so far neither of us have been hurt. It just means a call to our son, neighbor, or fire department to help me off the floor. This is embarrassing to me, but we continue to risk safety issues.

I am hesitant to call people to ask them to do anything for me or even just hang out with me. I don't want to have people come over because they pity me. I don't want to be a burden to anyone, while at the same time realizing I am quite a burden to Keith. My illness has changed my relationship with Keith's sister because I don't want to make her come over and assist me, as she did for her mother. My illness has complicated things between us. Of course, her main concern is for Keith's health.

I know that Keith's family is more emotional and comfortable talking about their feelings. I came from a different sort of family. While it's understood we love each other, we don't talk about emotions. I know my siblings love me and are concerned but don't know how to change the situation, especially since I live 200 miles away from them. (My sister lives even further away. We talk on the phone often but don't see each other but a few times a year. She still works as a school guidance counselor and is busy with her job.)

I accept our siblings as they are, but sometimes I don't understand the emotional aspect of Keith's siblings. I will say that Keith's father was always concerned about me, and kind. He treated me as if I were his very own daughter; I don't think he would want to "put me away" in a nursing home. He was one of the most loving and caring men I've ever known. On the other hand, Keith's mother thought I needed to be placed in a nursing home even while I was still walking and using my hands. She didn't want Keith burdened by a "handicapped" wife.

CHAPTER 25

TRIALS AND TRIBULATIONS

Keith:

It was 4:30 am when my phone went off and woke me. I wasn't sure if it was the alarm clock or Dare. Once I managed to open my eyes I noticed it was her calling. As I said earlier, Dare sleeps in her lift chair in the living room. If she needs something done, she calls through the Alexa program.

When I answered, she told me she needed to go to the toilet. I stumbled out of bed and went to give her relief. The arthritis in my back is worse in the morning, especially when I first get up. I usually have time to take my medications to help. However, this morning, like many, there wasn't time for the medication to take effect. I always get concerned that I'll drop Dare when lifting her out of her chair and placing her on the toilet. My balance and pain aren't good, but I refuse to spend 20 minutes wrapping a sling and lifting her. It's faster to take the risk even though it may be more dangerous.

Several years ago, we did have to call for help after Dare fell and I wasn't able to get her up. It was rather embarrassing when the big fire truck pulled up to the house and neighbors thought we were on fire. It took three men struggling to get her off the floor.

Dare is so afraid we'll need to call them again, and she would like to hide when the truck turns the corner to the house. We've had to call the fire department on a few occasions over the years. Twice when her chair got stuck after going off the sidewalk into some mud. Another time when I locked her into the car at the Board of Elections and she couldn't use hands to unlock the door!

When she was finished using the toilet, I placed her back into the lift chair where she could return to sleep. Since I was awake and she had found relief, I decided to go to the gym and try some stretching to get my back functional. The gym is open 24 hours, so I was able to arrive by 7am. While there, I got a call from a friend who was going for his regular walk at the park. He religiously walks every morning for exercise and stress management. I've not been able to walk the five miles in a while due to my back situation, but since I have better motivation, I decided to join him. We walked about a mile before I wasn't able to keep the pace and needed to stop. After all, I still needed to return home to dress and feed Dare.

Upon arrival home, Dare was awake and said she needed to use the toilet again. I went to retrieve the bedside toilet and placed it next to the lift chair for better transfer. She asked me if the pain patch was still in place on her buttocks where she had severe pain from a skin breakdown. I checked and told her it was missing. Luckily, I had another with which to replace it. As we discussed earlier, skin breakdowns easily lead to infection, creating the need for continuous preventative wound care patches. Dare has had several breakdowns, so the skin is very fragile and causes discomfort when sitting. She must often move her chair or have me adjust her position to get relief from the pain.

These are struggles of daily caretaking. This morning was one of those few times Dare became emotional accepting her condition. As I replaced the pain patch, she was in tears. These times are few and mostly containable. However, the weight of the day-to-day struggle had hit her. Lately, her inspiration and courage can turn into despair and discouragement. I think we've both had our moments and asked God for relief and help.

Dare questions why this is happening to her, and what "good" is she. She feels she is a burden to me and recently apologized for what she feels this disease has caused.

She wonders why several friends have died while she is still on earth, unable to hold her grandchildren.

I tried to encourage her, telling her she's an inspiration to many. I don't see how anyone could function the way she has. It must be extremely discouraging to sit in a chair all day, unable to use her hands or walk, and rely on someone to even scratch an itch. She told me that she had a lunch scheduled with a teacher with whom she had taught several years ago. She was to meet at 12:30.

It was disheartening for me to see Dare in a state of despair this morning. I know moments of frustration and pain are present at times for both of us in dealing with this disease. Again, it's normal to have these times, but we somehow find the strength to fight back and get up again. I attempted to point out her positive and inspirational attitude, and how many have commented on the blessings and encouragement they've received in her presence.

I dried her tears, dressed her, and applied her makeup (I've learned to apply eyeliner, eyebrows, and lipstick!). After activity, I fixed her breakfast by cutting and feeding her the food. She felt better and was ready to venture out.

Dare:

I often suffer from insomnia and have tried a multitude of methods to resolve this issue: Ambien®, Trazodone, Seroquel, TYLENOL® PM, melatonin, muscle relaxers, and meditation music. No matter what, I still often don't sleep more than two hours at a time. I'm still searching for what will help me sleep through the night. Friends have suggested medical marijuana, gummies, or brownies. If it becomes legal in North Carolina, I'll try this suggestion.

I have a weird chemical reaction to medications. I've awakened in the middle of surgery to hear surgical staff talking and the surgeon placing stitches. I once had Mohs surgery for some skin cancer on my nose. The doctor needed to go to a deeper layer and I started feeling pain. He said I should be numb for another 45 minutes, but I told him, "I can feel the pain," and he had to give me more medication. Another time, when I was doing an MRI, the doctor prescribed valium. I didn't feel any affect from the medication, even after taking three pills.

Another time home health treated me for a bed sore, and the hydrocodone prescribed did nothing for the pain. The doctor then prescribed oxycodone, which only held off the pain for three hours at a time instead of the usual six. I was in terrible pain, so he allowed me to take the medication every three hours. However, I then became constipated with projectile vomiting. I had to have an enema to relieve the constipation.

One other time after having LASIK eye surgery, I was promised I would "sleep like a baby" when I got home. That night I was still wide awake at eight o'clock. I called the eye doctor's nurse, who told me, "Out of thousands of patients, you are the first who hasn't been knocked out." It's a frustrating situation, not knowing until "the deed is done" what kind of reaction I'll have to a medication. It appears they go through my system quickly, which results in not being able to stay asleep. I'm still on the quest for a good night's sleep.

The older we get, the more relaxed we are with our morning routine, and it's nice not needing to be anywhere by a certain time. Sometimes I have a late breakfast and another meal later in the day. We each enjoy time to ourselves. Sometimes Keith goes to a back room while I listen to music. The Alexa device has made it possible for me to control the lights, change TV channels, make telephone calls, play games, and feel a little more independent.

I have a cat who cuddles in my lap, and we enjoy the silence together. I'm grateful I don't need to have Keith beside me every minute of the day. I am sure he enjoys it as well. He is my best friend but we both need our separate times.

I do appreciate what he does for me. It is not easy for anyone. I am grateful that I have as much as I do have and try not to focus on the losses. I prefer to focus on the positive. Keith and I hope that by writing this book it may help others in similar situations. We've tried to be honest. It is not always a dream life; sometimes it feels like a nightmare.

But each day we make a conscious decision to have the best day possible.

CHAPTER 26

PLACEMENT

Keith:

One of the hardest discussions Dare and I continue to have is planning for future care. I realize we need to stay in the present moment and not focus on future trouble but planning for future care is also important. We both know that her illness is one of continued progression. As we both age, there may come a time where I'm no longer able to undertake the physical demands.

While we have looked at various options available, the truth is the financial costs for care are overwhelming. In addition, Dare wants to stay in our home and would like to continue with the care provided. We've had to discuss the possible need for a placement in a nursing facility, especially if my health declines and/or I die. I'm concerned about what will happen to her. She believes she'll be able to hire help and continue remaining at home. This may be available for a period, but in reality, her financial resources may not meet the increased medical expenses.

We have had hard discussions on whether placement needs to happen now. Again, our healthcare system doesn't allow Medicare to cover these costs. She doesn't qualify for Medicaid without a major disruption in her retirement pension and social security, which then affects my ability to remain in our present circumstances.

In discussing our care needs, Dare feels that I (and my family) want to place her in a home. I know their discussion of placement comes from their concern for my health and abilities. My siblings have noticed, and are concerned for, the stress caused from demands being placed on me in caring for her at home. I would like to think my top priority is keeping her at home, even though my stress levels, at times, need an attitude adjustment!

In addition, the idea that a facility can give her the same kind of care and attention while allowing me to simply visit or take her out daily sounds great...but isn't realistic. I've worked in a hospital setting and referred patients to these facilities. I've had first-hand experience evaluating nursing homes. I know there are many staff members who try to do their best, but most CNAs are asked to handle eight to twelve patients on their shifts, preventing them from giving adequate levels of attention. Patients often wait long periods of time before their basic needs are met.

I realize that for many, placement is the only option under difficult circumstances despite the level of guilt. I am not being judgmental if that is the decision a family needs to make. The best many can do is make the most informed decision possible, then keep close tabs on the situation, and advocate for the loved one.

Most nursing facilities are expensive. Medicare is available for a limited time, but families are left with the financial burden if Medicare doesn't cover the expense. Most patients only qualify for Medicaid coverage after their assets have been exhausted. Because Dare has a monthly retirement pension and social security, she is currently "over the limit" and can't qualify for Medicaid without major changes to our living situation.

We do have a 401(k) plan and some investments, if needed at a later point. However, it may be that my health will also deteriorate to the point where both of us will need these investments to cover our costs. So there is major reluctance to spend that money now when we might need those resources later. It's depressing that, because people are living longer (even though they might be in a deteriorating state), most elderly are not able to obtain the care they need or deserve.

Dare and I realize the difficulty of our situation. We want to live in the moment, yet we also know our needs for a higher level of care will grow.

Dare:

My preference is to stay in our home, if possible, even if Keith precedes me in death. I am smart enough to know that, should my plan to live alone and utilize as much help as I can backfires, I would of course explore other options. But I don't believe in saying that things are impossible until all options are explored.

If I were to die first, I don't want Keith to doubt whether he took the best care of me that he could. I've told Keith I want him to find another love. He's devoted his life to me and deserves to be happy. I tell him that maybe he can find a young person to take care of him! He says, "No thank you. With my luck, she would have a stroke the day after we marry, and I would be in the same situation!" Truly Keith has been the love of my life. I'm sad this situation has forced him into this role. I couldn't be more blessed by this person to care for my needs.

CHAPTER 27

FINANCIAL COST

Keith:

One of the mistakes we made was never thinking that an illness like MS could occur, nor understanding the huge costs that awaited after an illness was diagnosed. While we've been blessed to have medical coverage for much of our treatment costs, there have been significant out-of-pocket expenses. And because we didn't have long-term disability coverage in place beforehand, we've had to pay out of our own pocket for many of the needed resources over the years.

It would have helped to have long- and short-term disability insurance policies to cover the multitude of out-of-pocket costs incurred for Dare's illness. If we had carried long-term insurance beforehand, we wouldn't have borne nearly the same level of enormous financial burden, and future long-term care in a residential or nursing facility would now be possible. But disability insurance isn't available after the fact.

When Dare was first diagnosed with multiple sclerosis, we did try – and fail – to obtain disability coverage. She was denied because we were honest and reported her new diagnosis.

One never knows when you might be faced with an illness, serious or not. A recommendation I now suggest is to make sure you always have both short- and long-term disability insurance along with regular health insurance…and to do so while you're healthy. Once you're diagnosed with an illness, it's too late to get coverage. The same can go for life insurance policies, which are also nearly impossible to get once you are diagnosed with a major illness. Most people have the option of buying this type of coverage through their employer. Purchase options are also available outside of employment, although they're usually more expensive. The expense of the premiums is nothing compared to the out-of-pocket costs one will sustain without it.

At this point, any long-term residential care costs we incur will have to be private pay. Neither private insurance nor Medicare will cover long-term residential placement. And Dare doesn't qualify for Medicaid without also losing her pension.

How much does a chronic illness cost?

We estimated the cost of Dare's illness over the past
25 years, and the figure is astounding: somewhere in
excess of $906,700. This includes an estimated $620,000
of medical costs paid by health insurance – their portion
of the doctor visits, lab work and diagnostic tests (MRIs,
x-rays, etc.) hospitalizations, medical rehabilitation
facilities, and medication (including her chemotherapy
drugs, the Avonex drug, steroid IVs, etc.). This figure
also includes around $286,700 we've paid…on our own.
Imagine how we could have used that money otherwise!

We attempted to break down these out-of-pocket
expenses that were outside of insurance coverage from
these 25 years. This list only covers the major items; the
smaller costs are just too numerous to even contemplate.

Medications

Avonex:	$25,200
25 years of medications:	$17,189
Alternative and integrative medicine doctors:	$1,345

Daily in-home skilled help

20 years before Keith retired:	$120,390

Physical Therapy

Since the beginning:	$10,000
Therapeutic horseback riding (four years):	$1,800
Muscle stretching therapy to prevent atrophy:	$3,120

Medical miscellaneous

Medicare Part B Premiums:	$23,856
Respite care costs:	$4,910
Corrective vision surgery (100% out-of-pocket):	$5,000
Surgery to insert port (out-of-pocket portion):	$1,400

Vehicles

Three special handicapped vans over the years (all used):	$36,000
Purchase and installation of a lockdown system to secure chair:	$4,800
Hand controls which allowed Dare to drive:	$900

Manual Wheelchair

Before the need for a motorized chair, Dare used a standard, manual wheelchair. This cost $500 out of pocket. Over the years we purchased multiple seat cushions to prevent skin breakdown for a cost of $900.

Motorized Power Chairs

Three-wheeled scooter:	$849
Three motorized chairs:	$6,800

(Our copayment after Medicare paid the bulk of the cost. Medicare replaces a chair every five years.)

Power Lift Chair/Recliners

One new chair:	$2,400
One used chair:	$350
One used chair:	$209

Miscellaneous Equipment

Standing table (rental):	$155
Walking Cane:	$16
Gait Belt for Walking:	$13
Three sets of reachers:	$63
Sliding board (for transfer from wheelchair to bed):	$40
Dumb bells and resistance bands:	$100
Gym membership:	$1,200
Two shower chairs:	$780
Two bedside toilet chairs:	$300
Shower bench:	$150
Lifts: one motorized:	$7,400
one used, portable Hoyer:	$90
Ramps: two exit ramps:	$1,400
one tractor ramp (for emergency	

exit use in the van):	$90
One replacement hospital bed:	$900
One power bed lift:	$1,344
Foot Braces (AFO):	$1,300
Two pairs of shoes to fit AFO:	$120

Travel Costs (gas/hotel/meals)

Charlotte MS Treatment Center:	$659
Atlanta MS Center:	$2,490

Mental Health Therapy

Stress management:	$1,224
Individual therapy:	$432

The estimated total out-of-pocket costs: $286,684. These are the out-of-pocket expenses we've been able to track over the 25-year period since Dare's diagnosis. There are certainly a multitude of other expenses we've forgotten or left by the wayside.

Our closest estimate of costs paid by health insurance:	$620,000

GRAND TOTAL:	**$906,684**

Dare:

We don't typically dwell on the cost of out-of-pocket expenses for my illness. Little good comes from discussing the issue except to illustrate the toll it's taken in our lives. Think how this money could have been spent otherwise! We're grateful we've been able to afford the care we've needed.

CHAPTER 28

PLANNING FOR
END OF LIFE

Keith:

Death is an extremely uncomfortable topic for me to accept, much less talk about. While there have been many hardships and struggles, I've never wanted to accept that one of us will be left alone to grieve. If I die before Dare, how will she meet her physical limits and demands? While we have some financial security for the future, I'm concerned there won't be enough.

As I mentioned, I worked in a hospital setting where many of my patients were placed in facilities due to their medical conditions, lack of family support, safety concerns, or inability to afford the costs of remaining at home.

I don't want Dare to face the stress of making end-of-life decisions alone. To avoid this issue, we've had discussions on this topic and have worked on final preparations for both of us. We've made lists of things that need to be taken care of: End-of-life decisions and documentation to ensure our desires and final wishes are carried out. Our will, health care power of attorney and living will documents. Our completed obituaries. All the necessary documents on file with the medical department and physician offices.

In addition, I've had open discussion with my doctor on the options available for a variety of scenarios. Dare has purchased grave sites at her home community church with a joint headstone (she also purchased a headstone for our child, Anna). Dare is working hard to organize her pictures and writing. She wants to have her business in order before the disease progresses further. She also wants me to be proud of her clutter being organized!

Initially, I was protective of Dare and didn't want to leave her with this task. I opted to appoint a friend to carry out my wishes and make medical decisions incorporating input from the medical team, Dare, and my family. However, on further thought, I realized that because she and I have been together for so many years, there is no one but my spouse better able to make those decisions.

Dare agrees with this plan.

Dare is often accused of being in denial about her situation and disease. Yet how can one be in denial when she's lived it every day? When she struggles every day to maintain a strong attitude? As I've said, I believe we have done an exceptional job fighting and dealing with the limitations brought to us as a result of illness given our situation. Yes, there are times of sadness, tears, despair, discouragement, and anger.

However, there are those times of connection, love, dedication, and faith that see us through. I have my struggles and moments of wanting to run away. But I don't think I could ever come to the place where I could leave the lady I love. I have gained much in the strength and love we've created through the hardships, pain, struggle, and hurt. I am grateful and appreciative for the times we've shared.

Many people may think that nursing home placement is the best decision for Dare. However, if either one of us meets the criteria for hospice care at the end of life, I would instead elect to utilize a residential hospice facility. I've worked at these facilities and know the excellent quality of care given to patients at the end of life.

If Dare dies before me, I have retirement money resources that she's m̲a̲ [...] ble. In addition, I have social security and 401([...] e. The question remains as to whether these fina[...] urces will offer the care we prefer. We may have to opt for placement in a facility, but are determined to have more of a say about how we wish to live at the end of life.

My career taught me the need for planning. I've often seen how the spouse or family members are left to make difficult decisions after a death. I've obtained a resource that helps plan at the end of life. This document addresses many of the considerations we've discussed, and provides information and instructions on what to include: names, addresses, phone numbers, contact information for physicians and attorneys, bank account numbers, investment account numbers, and information on our computer and phone passwords.

And of course, we've made decisions around cremation, burial site, and tombstone at Dare's home church in memory of our life together. We are members of a local church and have planned our funeral service.

CHAPTER 29

SELF-CARE SUGGESTIONS AND TIPS

Keith:

Whether you're a current caregiver or anticipate being one in the future, there are a range of personal physical and emotional challenges you can expect to encounter during your caregiving journey. Caregiving can result in love, satisfaction, and joy. But it also involves frustration, anger, anxiety, depression, and isolation...often at the same time! The wise caregiver will learn to identify those components before they become crisis points and have strategies in place to cope in a healthy way before stress and burnout take over.

Burnout is the state that occurs when a caregiver neglects their self-care to the point of mental and physical exhaustion and there are literally no internal resources left to give. When in the midst of their role, caregivers too often put their own self-care behind that of others. Any attention they give to themselves – respite, nutrition, and rest – comes too late.

Self-care is not selfish. It's the realization that one cannot continuously perform in this role without also attending to their own mental, physical, and spiritual needs and restoring a sense of balance. There are many strategies to avoid burnout, and the healthy caretaker learns to implement a regimen of practices that helps increase relaxation, foster self-esteem, and shift focus beyond the caretaking role.

Daily Routines

It's not hard to worry about the future, and it does take practice and awareness to remain focused in the present. Self-care in this capacity includes practicing meditation, yoga, breathing, or relaxation strategies. All of these can calm energy in the moment and definitely help to relieve stress when one starts dwelling on future troubles.

First among these is the conscious cultivation of daily positive thoughts and enjoyable activities, which shore up a caretaker's resilience to perform daily care routines. These daily moments can include listening to music, playing an instrument, taking a walk, meditation, massage, reading, or some form of sports. Chief among these is some form of exercise, which is perhaps the best way to manage stress and depression. It literally lowers the level of harmful chemicals in the brain. I've attempted to list (and practice) these activities to improve my own self-care and reduce stress.

Engaging in activities and tactics to avoid burnout and increase satisfaction is an individual choice. Self-care takes time, commitment, and follow-through, but the goal is to feel better and balance the physical, mental, and emotional frustration of caring for another.

When caretaking does become too much, it's easy to become prone to negativity and reactivity. One helpful practice I've found is to express negative emotions in a letter, writing about frustrations, demands, and problems. Of course, the letter is then destroyed or burned (not given to the loved one).

Respite Care
Respite care is a great self-care strategy and involves implementing physical time away from your loved one to rest and enjoy a change of scenery to reduce the negative impact of this role. The respite can be short or long – overnight, weekend, a week, or longer – and often

has multiple benefits for both parties in the caregiving situation: reprieve from each other, a refreshed sense of perspective, a renewed commitment to the task, and an opportunity to learn more about oneself and one's limits.

Some community agencies provide funding or scholarships for respite care, which can offset the costs. I recently took a respite week and spent it traveling to visit friends and relaxing a couple of days in a motel. I received a respite scholarship from the Council on Aging to be able to do this. And while this grant didn't cover all my expenses, it did fund the cost for a community health agency staff member who stayed and cared for Dare in my absence.

These healthcare agency folks are usually certified nursing assistants (CNAs) qualified to help with the daily routine of preparing meals, feeding, bathing, toileting, socialization, and even some house cleaning. They are not allowed to administer medication but can remind the person to take medication and may assist in placing medication in the mouth if the person is someone like Dare, who lacks the use of their hands.

Even if there is no community agency to help with the cost, I've paid money out of my own pocket for getaway time. Yes, it's costly for someone to stay with Dare, but not taking self-care respite time is costly to me. The money is always well-spent. To defray the costs, sometimes a trusted friend or relative may be willing to take the job. (This is a service I've also recommended church groups offer, provided they have a strong volunteer program.)

Another option is using an area nursing facility for short-term respite when other resources aren't available. There are several nursing homes in our area that offer respite care, provided they have open beds. Dare stayed in one such facility for a week while I was away.

Another suggestion for a shorter respite is the use of an adult daycare program, often provided by community agencies. These programs offer activities, supervision, and socialization for participants with a variety of needs. They provide meals and have a nurse available for medical needs. Case managers or discharge planners at the hospital may be a good resource for finding adult day programs in the community, along with access to other local services.

Again, coverage for this expense may be provided by scholarships, VA services, or community agencies, along with individual private-pay. While we haven't utilized the adult daycare in our community, I did have the opportunity to work as an interim program director in my past position at the hospital. I saw how well they work to fill a valuable need.

Sometimes close family and friends may be available to "staff" a respite. Dare's friend, Doris, will stay overnight with her while I'm gone. In addition to providing company, she involves Dare in activities I wouldn't normally like: grocery shopping, browsing thrift stores, and trips to the library. Eating out is something Dare really enjoys, and she and Doris have several favorite restaurants they both like to visit. Doris learned to operate our handicapped van so they can go to the mall, medical appointments, or shop outings.

Doris was first introduced to us through the Home Helpers agency we employed for bathing, and provided this service until she retired. She and Dare developed a deep friendship over that time. And although the agency had a non-compete policy prohibiting employees from working with their clients after leaving, Doris offered to help without being paid. Doris' friendship has been invaluable to both of us in helping with the overflow of errands, cooking, toileting, and other personal needs when I was still working.

I have personally found it effective to schedule a respite about every six weeks. In addition to the face value of time away, I find that having a regular respite on my calendar gives me something positive to look forward to. I know not taking this time can be dangerous in leading to burnout, frustration, and anger. I've told myself how important respite time is. I realize if I don't stick to a schedule, I will see a corresponding increase in irritation, stress, and anger.

Other Resources for Caregiving Support

As we've discussed earlier, there are many health care agencies that offer a menu of in-home services for pay. These services may include bathing, dressing, feeding, meal preparation, and some medical help. The agencies staff CNAs who are certified nursing personnel trained to deal with issues such as ours. The cost varies, but ours is usually $20 per hour. They can be scheduled for as many days or hours as needed, usually with a minimum number of hours of service.

Dare and I have used a home care agency for bathing. We also used their services as part of a respite program helping me take time away from caregiving duties. You can find home care agencies listed online and in phone directories. Community programs such as United Way, Council on Aging, and Interfaith Ministry either offer services or can often connect to those community resources and lists.

There are many community programs and resources available to assist with care. For example, our local Council on Aging offers a Meal on Wheels program. Volunteers deliver hot lunchtime meals to homebound residents (which can be frozen and re-warmed). This is generally a free service, but dependent on financial donations as part of their program.

Thanks to the pandemic, many grocery stores now offer shopping, where one can order online and have groceries delivered. Or you can order and pick up the groceries "curbside." We have used this service, and it cuts down on time and saves energy. Our favorite restaurants offer curbside service (and delivery, which is more expensive) of favorite meals. A newer offering is the variety of online meal kits one can order, and the food is quite good. Some kits have meal ingredients that one needs to prepare from scratch; others have meals ready to cook in the microwave or oven.

When it's needed, medical equipment can be obtained through a variety of resources. In addition to purchasing items (like a bed with lifting head and feet, or a handicapped van with a ramp) we've accessed items from a medical "loan closet" for medical supplies. The loan closet has things like toilet seats, hoyer lifts, hospital beds, canes, and crutches, to name a few. These items are generally for things needed on a short-term basis (after a surgery, for example) and available for a two-month loan.

Lastly, I know asking for help from friends and family is often hard. I feel like a burden when asking others for assistance. However, I'm also learning that many want to assist, but don't know how to ask. I have lists of tasks these individuals can do. For example: cooking an evening meal, running errands, or doing household duties.

Dare:

Respite is a good outlet for both caregiver and the recipient. I've enjoyed the times when Keith has gone for a respite break, if only for the change in caregivers. I prefer staying in my home, with friends or people from a home agency, to going somewhere else for respite. It's fun getting to know other people and having other experiences.

Staying focused in the present is so important. People need to remember that those who are in a chronic medical status are still "normal" people;

we're just navigating an abnormal situation. The illness does not defin son; it's only a part of the individual.

Having hobbies is a rewarding way to keep a positive attitude. Examples for me include doing jigsaw puzzles; reading books; listening to music or relaxation tapes; and sending cards to others for encouragement, birthdays, anniversaries, or get-well situations. Thinking of others is a great form of enjoyment.

My mother always said, "If you think your life is rough, just take a look around. There are many others who may be in a worse condition." I've taken her advice and found it to be so true. Attempt to be thankful for what you have. Count the blessings and focus on the positive gifts in life.

As my 99-year-old father tells me, "Each day is a good day. I made it through another day." I hope to be able to carry on with my father's outlook in life.

CHAPTER 30

GOOD SAMARITANS AND EARTH ANGELS

Keith:

On warm and sunny days, Dare still enjoys getting out of the house on walks, shopping, and luncheons, socializing with both friends and strangers she meets along the way. In visiting one of her favorite places – the local thrift shop – many kind people help open her doors, reach for items, and comment on her smile and attitude. They also give her encouragement, telling her how much of an inspiration she is to them and complimenting her spirit. Often people laugh as she drives by on her motorized chair, bags filled with items and various treasures tied to the back. I've made the comment that she resembles a homeless bag lady carrying her belongings down the streets. She's told me that her trips to town and the thrift shop are ways she entertains herself while I work.

Dare and I have met many of these good Samaritans and "earth angels" along our path. From the very beginning, these earth angels reached out in support, service, assistance, and love. When we've felt alone in our journey, it has been a gift to remember these special people. Dare and I are amazed at the number of loving and supportive citizens and strangers who've given many of these gifts. We realize we are fortunate to live in a small community where others hear of needs and respond accordingly.

Dare has always been highly active in many projects. She not only taught special education to disabled students but spent time encouraging and supporting children and their school activities.

Several years ago, Dare learned to write with her left hand. She always had an interest in writing and attended a creative writing class at our local community college. As a result of that class, she met several people and formed a writing group which came to our home weekly to write stories and poetry and provide critique for each other. There were roughly seven or eight individuals who came every week for over 15 years. One of the older men, Howard, would take Dare's stories and type up her notes, spending time to ensure her writing reflected exactly what she wanted said. He would drop them off each week before the group meeting to make any changes she wanted. The group was sad when Howard and his wife left the area and moved to Ohio.

Another member of the group, Marian Gowan, stepped up and offered to type for Dare. She also volunteered to help with communication needs, pay bills, and organize Dare's materials. Although she and her husband moved out of state after several years of providing this support, she continued to type up special projects that Dare needed by mail. In this way, Dare continued to actively write and publish her work in various articles, books, and magazines.

When Dare first started chemotherapy in Atlanta, we attended a church where one of the members organized a group of volunteers willing to serve a six-week rotation of support in our home. These individuals came once a week to assist in grocery shopping, house cleaning, laundry, and errands. We had one lady in her sixties who came to do cleaning and ironing. Due to her faith in God, Ms. Francis spent 12 years coming each week to help! She stated that this was her way of serving and she looked forward to spending the time with Dare. She was also a strong proponent of prayer and gave Dare the gift of being her prayer warrior. Dare would give her a list of needs from other people needing prayer as well, and Ms.

Francis would take these requests to a group of women who would offer prayer to God for assistance.

Several years ago, I received a telephone call from a friend who was active in a Sunday school class Dare and I had attended some 26 years ago. He reported that a group from this same class had heard the story of Dare's illness and my role as her primary caregiver. Several members of this class then formed a group with a service focus and wanted to do something for us. After some discussion, they decided to rotate a lunch time for Dare so I wouldn't have to come home from work to cook. This group has performed this service for the past five years, becoming good friends with Dare as a result. They report that they get as much enjoyment from their visits as Dare gets from of their companionship.

Dare is also eligible to receive Meals on Wheels through our local Council on Aging nonprofit, which furnishes lunch Monday through Friday. This has been a great service, especially when I used to work and didn't have time for a hot meal. If I'm not able to feed her the meal, we usually have someone who can assist.

There was a lady working in the school system who arranged for a local boarding home to prepare and deliver evening meals to our house. She also arranged to have a lady come over to wash and cut hair. This saved Dare from having to be transported out to have this done.

Men from a community leadership group built a ramp to provide better access to our home. We have had community, church, and civic groups offer financial support for needed equipment. One such community group, the Council on Aging, obtained a grant to provide "respite scholarships" to hire care for Dare while I take respite time to recharge my physical and emotional batteries. They also helped in the purchase of a lift chair with vibration and heat features to enhance circulation needs.

Family members have assisted in purchase of larger items such as a handicapped van with ramp. Without this van, we would not be able to attend medical appointments, grocery shopping, outings, etc. Family members have also helped in the financial cost of a lift to access the toilet and bathtub.

Another positive activity for Dare has been the ministry she provides for our church. Through the help of volunteers, Dare sends birthday greetings, anniversary cards, and letters of support and encouragement to all members of our church. So often those members later come up to Dare and thank her for her expression of care, love, and support. One Sunday, the minister used Dare as an example, saying she always asks for prayer for others, but seldom focuses on herself. Her spirit of giving to others is evident and sincere. She says she receives as much encouragement and support from others as she provides support to them.

These are but a few examples of the kindnesses, both given and received, as we continue to deal with this illness. We hope others dealing with hard circumstances can look at the blessings and gifts they receive from others.

Dare:

I've met many amazing people who, in one way or another, encouraged me, helped me, and made my life much better. The people in the thrift store that Keith mentioned have a restaurant next door. The profits from both their programs go to support battered women and children who need a safe environment. I've never regretted any of the money spent there. My best childhood friend and college roommate was the victim of a murder-suicide at age 41 by her boyfriend. She was so vibrant; it was tragic how her life ended. I therefore have a special place in my heart for women who are seeking safety from abuse.

It's hard for me to name every person who has come into my life because of MS. It warms my heart constantly, even the small kindnesses given. For example, I've had home agency helpers who have become good friends outside of their duties. One such person, Doris, used to be my bath lady. Even though she's retired from the agency, she still takes me on outings to the library, cooks meals, goes to the grocery, and helps me send correspondence. She takes my cat to the vet, cleans the litter box, and stays with me when Keith goes on respite. She automatically sees what I need and responds, doing such things as providing range of motion to my arms and legs, before I ask. We always have a great time and I appreciate her friendship.

My next bath lady, assigned after Doris left the agency, stays after performing her duties to help me organize pictures and write letters. Due to the pandemic, she wasn't able to work with me, but stayed in touch by phone.

Another helper, who only spent about three hours with me, came by at Christmas and gave me a gift certificate for $100. She had received extra money from another client, thought of me, and simply wanted to share her blessings. She and I both also connected over recipes, so she came by one day and brought me a recipe book.

Through our circumstances, Keith and I have met so many caring and supportive individuals. Keith calls these good Samaritans "earth angels." Last week, for example, I bumped into a lady I've known for more than 30 years but hadn't seen in quite a while. We stopped and caught up with each other's lives, and she asked if she could say a prayer for me. I said yes, and she said a prayer for me, right then and there. I cannot tell you how many times strangers have stopped to ask if they could give a prayer, and I always accept any prayer they offer. I do feel I meet these people for a reason, and they create the moments for which I am most grateful.

I believe in earth angels and good Samaritans, whether I've known them for two minutes or two decades. One day a homeless man in the library offered to turn the pages in the newspaper for me to read. I often think of Jan the RN, who was with me at Anna's death to give me such deep care and support. She was a perfect stranger who made such a difference in my life. So, when I see a person who needs encouragement, I hope to be an "earth angel" and find some tiny way to support them as well. We can all be kind to each other. You don't need to be rich to bring brightness into someone else's life.

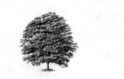

CHAPTER 31

FAITH AND ATTITUDE

Keith:

Faith has played a significant part in my caregiving role. It has always been a part of my life but seems to have strengthened since Dare's illness. I have often prayed for strength to carry on when circumstances and fears have taken over. There are times I feel closer to God; I don't always understand His plan but rely on faith that there is a reason. This faith gives me strength.

I remember an episode which happened during my early years in graduate school. One afternoon when I was walking home from class I had one of my many conversations with God, asking for a sign of His existence. I walked a few feet and found a marble on the side of the walkway. I thought it was interesting and, while I'm not sure if this was the sign I looked to receive,

I took notice and placed it in my mind.

The next afternoon, I again asked for a sign. And again, I found another marble a few feet away. I found myself wondering if this was the message that He existed. I remember sharing this story with Dare, who just looked at me with questioning eyes. Several days later, we were walking on campus when we had a disagreement and walked away from each other angry. Several minutes later, she came back with a smile on her face. She opened her hand and showed me the marble she found. She felt it was a sign from God saying, "I'm on your side." We both laughed and I said, "Yes, He must be!"

Several months later, we walked down a country road in Hendersonville, questioning whether or not we wanted to move back to the mountains after I finished my graduate studies. A few feet later, we found a black marble half buried in the dirt. It had obviously been there for some time, but we took it as God saying, "Yes!" Shortly after, we made the move back to Asheville, N.C.

The first day Dare went to a new teaching job, nervous and anxious, she opened her car door and found a marble on the ground. She took this as a sign she was in the right place.

When we took our daughter, Elizabeth, to Appalachian State University for orientation, we were anxious about leaving our first-born at college. As I rolled Dare across campus, she suddenly said, "STOP, roll my chair back!" And there on the pavement was a multi-color marble, a sign that she would be fine, in God's care.

Marbles have played a significant part during times of decision making. To us they are a sign of affirmation. However, the most significant marble episode was when I agreed to do a mental health home visit with a lady who was disabled and could not come to my office. This was the only time I agreed to do a home visit. When I entered the home, she had a jar of marbles on her coffee table. I stated that she must collect marbles. She replied, "These marbles belonged to my twin boys, who were killed in an automobile accident. I keep them on the coffee table to remind me of them."

When riding home that same afternoon I passed the graveyard where Anna was buried. I noticed the flowers on her grave had been blown over by the wind. I stopped to straighten them and saw a crystal-clear marble at the head of her tombstone. I returned home and said to Dare, "Anna is in God's hands!"

Most people hearing this story would say that we've lost our marbles! But to this we would say that we have learned to place God closer in our lives. I know the caregiving role is difficult, but I'm learning to be more grateful for what God has given me. I continue to pray for commitment, awareness, and trust in His plan.

I have grown in my faith over the years. I trust that God loves me, and I don't have to be perfect to be in His care. I know His blessings and my faith have carried me through times of frustration and struggle in my caregiving. Dare's faith also gives me hope and encouragement. There are times I want to run away, but I'm called back to carry on with my responsibilities. I have often asked for forgiveness for the times of discouragement and wanting to give up. We both have been through hard times but have also been equally blessed by the gifts and opportunities that provided strength.

Dare:

My home church, a congregation of about 80 people, had a minister who only preached every other Sunday because we had to share him with three other small churches. Of course, we also had Sunday school, vacation bible school, and youth fellowship groups. When I was 11, I gave my life to Christ during a revival held at Lilesville Elementary school gym. In the 1960s, I didn't know any female ministers; it was an all-male occupation.

When my uncle became sick with melanoma, I totally believed God would cure him. I prayed and begged for his recovery, but my prayers were not answered. I was truly angry with God for about a year. I told Him every day, "You let me down. I trusted you to give him a miracle. Why did you let me down?" After that, I learned we must accept His will over ours. He may want to know the desires of our hearts, but as my mom said, "Sometimes His answer is 'No' and we have to learn to accept that."

I feel that my MS is part of God's plan. It is not what I would want for myself or anyone else, but I believe God will use it – and me – for some good purpose. I don't know exactly what this plan is, but I continue to trust in God. I know He will not leave or forsake me.

My faith is extremely important to me, and always has been, but I think since this illness I have had to depend on it more than ever. I'm not sure how people survive a chronic progression of an illness without having faith and love of family.

CHAPTER 32

GIFTS RECEIVED

Keith:

Recently, on a road trip with Dare, I asked, "So tell me, what, if any, are the gifts you've received as a result of your MS? In other words, are there things or people who have given you certain lessons or insight into your disease?"

Dare:

It didn't take me long to answer Keith. One of the best – and most important – gifts received from MS has been learning to live in the present. I've never been one to live in the past, but I was bad about projecting into the future. I have learned to enjoy the present to the best of my ability.

My future is too scary and unknown. I came to realize it does me no good to worry about the length or quality of my life. With the diagnoses of MS and blood cancer I realize that each day is a gift, and I don't want to squander it with worry or dreams of the future. I am going to live for the present moment and not worry about tomorrow.

All we have is today. Tomorrow is not promised to anyone. It's important to appreciate the present and its gifts.

Another gift received has been the many kind people I have met along the way who've encouraged me. I thank God for my "earth angels" and for bringing them into my life. Many people have said I am an inspiration to them, but I don't recognize myself in this way. It's not me who is the inspiration, but God and the loved ones who stand by me in my time of need.

I am grateful to have my children grown and wonderful grandchildren thriving. I've met many people who touched my life and given prayers, encouragement, and support along our journey. I am thankful for the gift of my husband, who has stayed with me during these days to help with the daily challenges of meeting my needs.

Keith:

Dare continued pointing out that as most people live, they focus on goals, careers, transfers, and promotions. She says this disease has taught her these areas aren't the important components of life. The most important priorities are the love of God, faith, family, and loved ones.

Both Dare and I comment on the gift of humor. Many of our "earth angels" have understood the importance of humor and laughter. Without the ability to laugh, we would live in an incredibly stressful and depressive state. Often, we share humorous comments, tell jokes, make fun, or see things that give hope to others. I am very appreciative that I've developed the gift of humor; it helps me deal with the pressures of the task.

The gift of humor has certainly assisted us in the release of frustration and stress. We both have the ability to tell jokes, make fun, and better cope through the use of humor. I'm sure some people may be shocked by the things we may say, but they're said in order to break the stress of daily frustration. Humor makes the situation more tolerable. And having this sense of humor appreciated by my spouse and others gives us a sense of being together in this illness.

Here are several examples:

We took a trip to the beach and Dare wanted to find seashells along the oceanfront. We rented a special "PVC" wheelchair from the recreational department in Myrtle Beach. This is a lightweight plastic wheelchair specifically designed for the beach, with wheels that stay on top of the sand to make it more mobile. I went to pick this special chair up but found I couldn't fit it into our car. However, since our car was a convertible, I put the top down and literally held it by hand while driving down the highway, hoping it would stay in the car.

Further hilarity ensued when I placed Dare into the chair; it was so big that she looked like tiny Edith Ann from the TV show *Laugh In*. I spent the afternoon pushing this monster, picking up every shell she wanted and continuing down the beach. Afterward, the bottoms of my feet were cut from stepping on shells I couldn't see over the chair. When we returned to the hotel and pushed the chair up the sand bank, she said she had a "wonderful time" on the beach! I responded, saying, "I'm sure glad you did, but I'm exhausted!"

Another adventure happened when we went to a shopping mall. It was the first time we used a rented wheelchair. I didn't realize that when taking someone down a ramp, it's better to go down backwards. Not realizing this, I headed straight down the ramp from behind. Dare didn't have a seat belt fastened, and I ended up dumping her out of the chair onto the parking lot! Luckily, with her skirt up over her head, exposing her to the world, she was less hurt and just more embarrassed. We sat on the ground until I fixed her dress and laughed before we got up and on our way.

One afternoon, Dare was able to drive her power chair down the road to the eye doctor for an appointment. Of course, they dilated her eyes. When she left the office, she came to a curb on the sidewalk. Not being able to see clearly, she attempted to determine if she could negotiate this obstacle and jump the curb. There was an EMT ambulance driver stopped at a nearby red light. Dare spoke out and said, "Do you think I can jump this curb?" He said, "Go for it!"

Well, Dare did just that! And in the process overturned her chair, throwing her onto the ground. The driver and another man jumped out to assist her back into the chair. Dare was so embarrassed and said, "I can't go out again; I'm going to have to dye my hair!" During the incident, another lady called the police but Dare got back into her chair and got away before the police came. She thought she could escape the embarrassment, and nobody would recognize her. However, I reminded her that she wouldn't be too hard to identify once she was back in a power chair on the street. She just laughed.

When it was time for Dare to have a yearly mammogram, I needed to escort her. My job was to help lift her up and hold her so the machine could get a good picture. At one point, I had my head down toward her waist, trying to hold her tightly in place. One of the nurses asked her if she was ok. Before she was able to answer, I spoke out from below, "Yes, thank you, I'm fine!" Dare laughed so hard, knowing they had no concern for me but asking her if she was comfortable. Thank goodness it's come to the point where they no longer try to do a mammogram; they do an ultrasound test instead. No more holding her up!

One spring afternoon, Dare and I visited the grave of our daughter, Anna. It had rained that morning and the grass was wet. As Dare rolled her chair over the cemetery yard, she suddenly became stuck in the mud. She accelerated in an effort to loosen its grip, but instead flipped her chair backwards and found herself hanging upside down. As usual, not being hurt, I managed to push the chair back and pick her up from the ground as we laughed.

When taking a walk to town, we learned to place a jacket or pocketbook on her lap because the wind can suddenly blow her skirt over her legs, exposing areas that she would rather keep private. I've had to make more than one sudden dash to pull her skirt down.

One of the funniest stories (which may seem like dark humor to most) occurred at the funeral of a friend named Sarah. Sarah was only 50-plus years old and had died of multiple myeloma. Dare and I were sitting in the sanctuary when a former principal of Dare's sat next to her. As the service ended and they began to roll the casket up the aisle, this principal turned to Dare and said, "Dare, what can I do for you? I think of you often." Dare responded to her saying, "Just pray for me." The principle looked at Dare and said, "I do that every day for Sarah."

As if on cue, the casket came by our pew. Dare looked at the coffin, then back at the lady, and said, "Wait a minute, you pray for Sarah every day? On second thought, don't pray for me!" I just looked at Dare and broke out laughing.

One night we went to a John Denver music tribute. We had seen John in concert on three different occasions and loved his music. In fact, one time he stayed at the local hotel after giving a live concert in Asheville. When Dare and I spent the night in this same hotel later that year, we were told it was the same room John had stayed in. We would laugh and say we "spent the night with John."

At this same concert, we weren't able to dance like a normal couple, so I took over and danced with her in the wheelchair. Later that night, a gentleman came up to me and said how much he and his wife enjoyed seeing us dance. He could tell the love we had for each other, and it got him thinking of his own relationship with his wife. We've had many comments similar to this, as we've been able to maintain a strong connection. We connect with our eyes and hold on to those times of early intimacy in our relationship.

I play guitar and sing. There are several songs I've recorded over the years that she's liked. I can sing a song that brings up wonderful memories and strong emotions. She has always loved my playing, even though I might sing off key! Whether I sing on-key or off, Dare always compliments me and asks that I record more songs for her. Someday I might be so inclined to perform them.

When dealing with such a serious situation as a chronic, progressive illness where research hasn't yet developed a cure, we are left having to make the best of a hard situation. I am grateful for the times Dare and I can find humor or laugh in order to survive.

Dare's attitude and determination to make the best of her condition continue with an outward smile and high spirit as she's faced the challenges over the years. I'm amazed at how she's conducted herself and continues to show others that she's a strong and independent lady even while limited in some of her daily activities. Whether or not internal fears are present, she's not going to show loved ones a negative attitude toward the hardships faced.

Love is a short four-letter word with a big, broad meaning. It's the commitment described in the marital vows "for better or worse, in sickness or health." Our relationship is an overall gift of love which goes beyond the challenges. We have a history shared, children, grandchildren, financial stability, memories, and a devotion to maintain our commitment to the best of our ability.

CHAPTER 33

DARE'S OUTLOOK

Dare:

MS is just a part of my life. It is not my whole life. And I am much more than an MS victim. My mind is still active, which is both a blessing and a curse. I do have many interests and a desire to continue having a good life. I feel very blessed with my family, my husband, children, and grandchildren. They are the most important people to me. If they love me and still want me to hang around, I will fight to do so regardless of the illness or what may come.

I feel love and faith are the most important things in life. Sometimes I think it would be easier to give up, but I don't want to leave that kind of legacy to my children and grandchildren. I want them to know that life is not always fair, but it's our job to make the most of what we're given. I hope that when I die, my loved ones will carry on and not grieve too much for me. I can honestly say that I have had a good life, blessed with a good childhood and the love of my family.

I must speak to my faith now. I have always believed in God and his promises. This is a day-by-day journey and challenge, knowing my health is declining. Besides the MS, I've dealt with the blood cancer diagnosis for the past several years. I know that, at my age, I am looking more toward the end of my life. It's okay; I believe God will help me through the process. I just hope that I have left something good behind me.

As the years roll by, I accept that my health continues to decline, and the disease is unlikely to stop or reverse. I have been diagnosed for 25 years, have not walked for 18 years, and have lost the use of my hands for 12 years. I have been confined to wheelchairs for most of the years of my diagnosis. I have been through many treatments, including 29 months of chemotherapy, seven years of Avonex shots, IV steroids, blood draws, years of physical therapy, four seasons of therapeutic horseback riding for core strength, occupational therapy, and stress management therapy. I took early retirement from a job I loved because it was time to step aside. It wasn't fair to continue while there were eager and able-bodied teachers seeking employment. Plus, I needed to retire while I was still standing. I wanted to still feel valuable to the school and felt it was the right thing to do.

At first, I was leery of attending MS support groups. I didn't want my identity tied to being a victim of MS. I realize I have MS, but I'm not just MS. Therefore, I didn't wish to focus on the negative condition of the illness. At the first meeting I was nervous, thinking there would be a lot of crippled people in wheelchairs. When I walked into the room, no one was in a wheelchair. I returned years later to listen to a topic being presented in which I was interested. This time, when entering the room, I realized I was the crippled one in a wheelchair.

I didn't return after that because I didn't want others to see my deteriorating condition and become too frightened and depressed of their future. I've always been sensitive about providing a positive attitude and looking at my blessings. Yes, I have experienced loss, depression, shattered dreams, physical limitations, and isolation from activities I enjoy. But I still look toward God and my faith to make it through the hard times.

One of my major disappointments with MS has been not being able to care for my parents or Keith. Being five years younger than Keith, I thought I would be taking care of him and my parents. I've also grieved not being active with my grandchildren. I always looked forward to having my children, and being here with my grandchildren, doing special activities like cooking, driving to the park and zoo, visiting their homes, and babysitting. Instead, I feel everyone must take care of me.

When I lost the ability to use my hands, I was no longer independent to drive, write, turn the pages in books, put on my own makeup, dress, etc. Having even one functioning hand would give me more freedom to accomplish my daily activities. As it was, I was right-hand dominant and had to learn to use my left hand to do those activities. Then I lost function in that hand as well. That was a hard adjustment – not being able to dress or put on my own makeup. I could once drive my power chair with my left hand, but I no longer have the independence to shop or go to town on my own.

Keith continues to give me the care I need. He has been here so I can remain at home, even though I know there are times he would like to be free of the responsibility. I am grateful and blessed not to be in a nursing home, but to remain in my own home. I've had short stays at a nursing home, and know the staff tries to do their best providing care. But they are typically understaffed and not able to respond to things as quickly as one might need assistance. Often these homes advertise themselves providing quality care, but unless you have a family member or person to oversee the care given, it doesn't always happen as advertised.

People ask me if I am angry because of the illness and the many disappointments it's brought. The answer is no; I'm not angry. Things happen in life over which we have no control, and therefore need to accept. I am thankful for the blessings I've received in life. There are many who are miserable, angry, depressed, or negative in their circumstances. MS and a blood cancer diagnosis haven't been nearly as devastating as the death of my child, Anna.

Some may say I live in denial, but I say I am the one living with the effects of a crippling disease...how can I be in denial? I live this every day, every minute, of my life. I simply trust in God and know he will see me through. My husband, proves his love and devotion to me in a very and concrete way by taking on the constant caring for me.

We used to wonder, "What is love?" And now I know.

CHAPTER 34

REFLECTIONS

Keith:

It is strange how life presents challenges. Often one finds their way to a goal or a situation only to have everything change direction. I'm not sure how you see challenges or experiences, but over the years my pattern is to analyze, question, and learn lessons. That is not to say I've always had answers, but I look at ways to cope and adjust to the situation.

I didn't have special dreams of how my life would be during retirement years. There certainly are avenues and lessons learned from my struggle to be a caretaker for my partner. But I'm truly fortunate to have a good marriage, good children, and a career that supports my family. Like so many others, we were busy in the day-to-day activities of rearing a family, providing support and love to each other, and being with friends in our social activities and events. I have to say it has been a good journey overall. Count the blessings, see the glass half full.

However, with the many challenges we face there comes a time for reflection. As I've reached my 72nd year, I realize most of my life is behind me. I have completed many of my goals: rearing good children, spending time with my grandchildren, and caring for my wife. But I haven't done the best job looking at my own needs. This statement is not intended to focus on myself in a "selfish" sort of way, but to become more aware of my emotional, physical, and mental well-being, and finding balance in my role.

Being a caretaker, especially to a significant other, presents challenges different from most and raises many complicated issues. It hasn't been an easy journey, but like many, we do the best we can and make difficult decisions. It reminds me of a saying inscribed on my father's tombstone: "I did my best under the circumstances." I know how true that statement was in his life.

One Sunday morning our assistant senior pastor requested members to do a homework assignment on the word "surrender" and another on "His Will." So I've been thinking about the word "surrender." Surrender is hard for me to do; I've always tried to be in control, but surrender implies giving up control. I want to do it my way and not necessarily God's way. However, the more thought I give it, I realize surrender is not giving up, but allowing reliance on, and trust in, God's will.

People often ask how I cope with the responsibility as caretaker to a spouse who is dependent on me for every physical need. I say that many times the footsteps in the sand are truly those of Christ carrying me through the day. I am not meant to do this alone.

In John 3:30, the gospel says, "He must become greater and greater, and I must become less and less." An interpretation implies that the more I rely on God and give Him the glory, the less important I become in the struggles of caretaking. It's not all about me.

It's natural for us to want more control and forgo praising God for the benefits and blessings provided. In my moments of doubt, confusion, and questioning, I've asked why this situation happened, not only to me, but to such a wonderful spouse. I ask for help in accepting our situation. I know there are answers, but not necessarily in a timeframe that suits me. It is in His will, not mine. God has a plan. I may not understand but need to trust.

I now ask myself, "How do I want to spend whatever

time rema[...]n the past
decades, I [...] "survival"
mode that [...] routine we
often do n[...] we just do
what we'v[...] ealize that
I'm now p[...] come more
aware of h[...] e met so as
to better c[...] exploring
this proces[...]

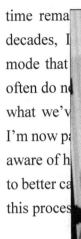

As I've sta[...] the past 25
years, I've [...] ve includes
commitme[...] illness has
impacted [...] ship, and
our love. Within its complexities and many conflicting
emotions and thoughts, I am committed to make the best
out of a difficult situation. It's what keeps hope and faith
alive.

Dare:

Our daughter, Elizabeth, has a favorite mantra: "What doesn't kill you makes you stronger." I think of this often as I reflect on our journey of the past several years. As my body gets weaker, other aspects of my life must become stronger in order to survive. I fight daily to keep this disease from taking my happiness, and my love of life and family. I don't want "it" to be the winner. I feel strongly that attitude and faith are 90% of the battle for anything. It's amazing how attitude can color everything.

CHAPTER 35

FUTURE CHANGES

Keith:

We are both uncertain of the future course of this disease. We realize that, as the progression continues, there will be further challenges to overcome. We plan to fight, and to work together to meet the unknown.

We choose courage and faith and laughter. Despite the challenges, frustrations, and difficulties we've faced over these past years, I'm also grateful for the gifts gained, people met, experiences given, love shared, children and grandchildren born. Regardless of this situation, I would marry her all over again! We have a connection that is hard to explain. From the special day we met, Dare has enriched my life and given me meaning and purpose.